Statistical Principles
in Health Care
Information

Statistical Principles in Health Care Information

Second Edition

S. James Kilpatrick, Jr., Ph.D.

Department of Biostatistics
Medical College of Virginia
Virginia Commonwealth University

University Park Press
Baltimore · London · Tokyo

UNIVERSITY PARK PRESS
International Publishers in Science and Medicine
Chamber of Commerce Building
Baltimore, Maryland 21202

Typeset by The Composing Room of Michigan, Inc.
Manufactured in the United States of America by Universal Lithographers,
Inc., and The Optic Bindery Incorporated.

Library of Congress Cataloging in Publication Data

Kilpatrick, S.   James, 1931–
    Statistical principles in health care information.

    Includes index.
    1. Medical statistics. I. Title.
RA409.K54 1977   362.1'01'5195   77-359
ISBN 0-8391-1107-X

Contents

List of Figures

List of Tables

Preface to Second Edition

The second edition of this book has benefited from the many reviewers who have criticized it in detail while recommending it to their colleagues. It is still intended for use by those in various health professions with problems of interpreting large data banks. Accordingly, it does not contain any additional nonparametric procedures other than those already contained in Sections 7.4 and 9.7.2.

This text recognizes that most analysts use a computer, and Section 12.6 describes one package of statistical programs as an example. The book tries to meet today's needs for reasonable expositions of statistical techniques now available through statistical programs. Accordingly, an additional chapter on forecasting, consisting of a traditional review of regression techniques and an elementary consideration of time series, is added.

To make this edition more useful, at the back of the book there is a list of definitions of new terms introduced in the text in boldface type.

I am indebted to a large number of people for improving this text. First, to those reviewers and others who have written to me pointing out inconsistencies and ambiguities. (Hopefully, all errors have been eradicated in this edition.) I am also indebted to my colleagues, especially Rochelle Ascher, for review, advice, and assistance in preparing the second edition.

The author was partially supported during the period of this revision by Grant 1 R01 HS 01899-01 from the National Center for Health Services Research, HRA.

Preface

This book is designed for readers who need a grasp of statistical principles in their health care professions, whether these be administration, practice, or research. It should also be of value to a wider audience because of its style. In general, statistics texts are either rigorous or nonrigorous. Rigorous texts depend heavily on mathematics, use an elaborate notation, and are unsuitable, therefore, for readers who need a basic knowledge of statistics but do not aspire to becoming statisticians. Books written for nonstatisticians tend to be either "cook books," in which the reader is shown how to carry out various statistical procedures without being given any explanation, or watered-down theoretical texts, in which the mathematics and notation are kept to a minimum and the material is presented theoretically.

This text is nonrigorous and attempts to introduce statistics by way of discussion and example. Often a statistical term is first used without an explicit definition: the meaning is to be derived from the context and the usual meaning of the word in English until the definition is given. The Contents and the Index should be helpful in this context. The notation used is reasonably standard, and the meanings of the symbols used are given in the Appendix.

No mathematical background is required of the reader, so this text is suitable as a first book in statistics, especially for those practicing in or intending to enter one of the health sciences or an allied health profession. On completion of this book the reader should be able to use one of the many "cook books" or to study an elementary theoretical text. Hopefully, this book will not be the reader's sole exposure to the subject. However, the book is intended to be self-contained and covers the major topics, texts, and applications of statistics.

A quick perusal will reveal how heavily the text relies on the *Documenta Geigy Scientific Tables,* seventh edition, which contains an excellent set of statistical tables freely adapted here for beginners. I am much indebted to the editors of *Documenta Geigy* for their permission to extract and to reproduce some of their tables.

Finally, I wish to record my indebtedness to my students and colleagues who pointed out errors and the misuse of "clearly" and other words in the manuscript. A special "thank you" goes to Shirley Carpenter for her devotion to the task of typing the manuscript and for the high quality of work she turned out.

To George Dockrell, Jack Spong, and many others who brought me to life.

1

Nature, Use, and Analysis of Hospital and Health Care Data

1.1 NATURE OF HEALTH CARE INFORMATION

Decisions in the management of hospitals and in the treatment of patients are made on the basis of information. This information may be subjective (the baby did not look well; the morale of the hospital employees is low) or objective (the baby's temperature is 101.8°F; the typical new employee resigns from his job after about nine months). This book deals exclusively with the latter type of information—objective, unemotional facts that can be checked by other people (auditors, physicians) and that can be communicated. For example, to say that a person is cyanotic implies personal judgment on what constitutes cyanosis (oxygen lack), but the statement that blood pressure is elevated can be made more precise by quoting the systolic and diastolic blood pressures, the method of recording these, and the norm or control values used.

This emphasis on the objective aspects of health care is not meant to diminish the importance of subjective information. Thus, Dr. Mendel Sheps, herself a statistician, has stated that a number may be precise but inaccurate while a description may be vague but accurate. Health care and health system administration are arts in which the "feel" of the case or system is very important even though it cannot be quantified. It is this subjective aspect of health care that leads many to maintain that the computer will never replace the physician in diagnosis. The physician cannot say how or why he arrives at a given diagnosis, for in doing so he uses all five senses and interacts with the patient as a person. No computer can replace the nurse's warm greeting or compassion. Nevertheless, a systematic structure for the use of objective facts has been developed, and it is this body of knowledge that is presented in the following chapters. Occasionally our objective facts will lead us to human situations; cold statistics can reveal subjective problems. A high personnel turnover rate, for example, may indicate low morale; a high incidence of requests for transfers from nurses may indicate an overly demanding supervisor.

A numerical item of information is called a **statistic**, and the term "descriptive statistics" therefore refers to a collection of numbers describing a system. The word **statistics** is also used to refer to the body of procedures that have been developed to process information. Thus "descriptive statistics" is different from the "theory of statistics" or "statistical inference," since the latter two terms refer to the procedures rather than to any body of information. The use of these terms should be obvious from the context.

The most important characteristic of health care information is *variation*: patients differ, illnesses manifest themselves in different ways, costs increase, duration of labor varies. However, this variation itself is apparently governed by certain laws which are described below. All health care information varies with respect to some norm or average. If we can deduce from a set of data, in which each reading represents an individual patient, what the "average" experience of these patients is and *also* describe the observed variation about this average, then we shall be in a better position to interpret future data of this nature than we would be without this overall view.

In this text, then, we are concerned with making the reader aware of variation in health care information and with showing how variation can be controlled and how conclusions that take this variation into account can be drawn. Too often the student is taught the norm or ideal and enters practice with concepts that, in the light of experience, are rapidly modified to allow for variation.

1.2 CLASSIFICATION OF INFORMATION

The subjective is generally indicated by "I think . . ." or "I feel . . ." or "In my opinion . . ." Subjective conclusions may be based on isolated objective facts. "My grandfather smoked cigarettes all his life and lived to age 92. How, then, can cigarette smoking be harmful?" In statistics we are interested not in the single fact, the single patient, the single hospital, or the single public health district, but in collections of objective facts about these items. We can use these bodies of information to predict the characteristics of single future items. For example, the prognosis for a woman with a given stage of breast cancer with no lymph node involvement who is treated radically is predicted from *past* information on similar patients. The knowledge that bed occupancy in a hospital is 80% is not of great value unless this fact is compared with the average bed occupancy for comparable hospitals in the same period.

For a given item of interest (say, hourly pay of nurses' aides), we can then have one value (the hourly pay of one aide), a number of values (the hourly pay of 36 of the 50 nurses' aides employed in the hospital), or all values (the hourly pay of all 50 nurses' aides employed in the hospital). These examples introduce the concepts of population and sample. A **population** is simply the total collection of items of interest, and the **sample** is a subgroup of this. In the above example, the population implied is the 50 hourly wages paid to the 50 nurses' aides employed at the hospital. (Note that a population does not have to be composed of people but can consist of some attribute of all items of interest.) A sample (the hourly wages of some nurses' aides) can vary in size from one to any number smaller than the size of the population. If the sample size equals the population size, it is called a **census**. The federal government enumerates the population every ten years in a census. If we were interested in age, we would have a population of over 200 million ages. A hospital might enumerate its inpatients at the same time that the federal census is taken and find that it contained 1501 inpatients of 1501 ages. From the point of view of the hospital, these 1501 patients constitute a population, but they may also be considered a sample of the total population of the United States. Strictly speaking, if we were interested in age only, we would consider the 1501 ages in the inpatient population as either a census (of the ages of inpatients in that hospital) or a sample of over 200 million ages of the total population of the United States.

1.3   TIME AND SPACE

Information should be qualified as describing certain periods and regions. Health care is dynamic both in time and space—people age, teeth decay, people change jobs, etc. We know, for instance, that a person's body temperature varies diurnally.

A hospital census will change from day to day. **Vital statistics** such as the death rate will change from year to year. Epidemics greatly affect **morbidity rates**. The population of interest should be specified clearly. It may be the white population of the United States or the residents of California. Often, in health care, we define a human population in terms of residence (living in a certain area) or in terms of receiving certain services (outpatients) or in terms of membership in certain groups (Medicare patients, college students, or employees). The mobility of the population in this country makes it very difficult to define the population served by a given hospital, health district, or family practice. These difficulties should never be obscured.

1.4   USE OF HEALTH CARE INFORMATION

Objective data in health care (birth certificate, death certificate, medical insurance claims) are of primary value to the individual in his dealings with the government, with the providers of medical care, and, as a patient, with respect to the effective diagnosis and treatment of his illness. These uses are well understood, and we will not elaborate on them further. In aggregate, these records serve to measure the health of a community or nation. Frequently, overall figures such as the **Infant Mortality Rate** are compared with similar figures from other nations in order to judge how well or poorly a nation is doing in the provision of health care. At the local level, data on the incidence of an infectious disease can alert a community to the dangers of an incipient epidemic and steps can be taken to avert the transmission of this disease. The hospital administrator may compare his average cost per patient per day with that of other hospitals or with a national average. The average waiting time for patients with nonacute conditions to be admitted to the hospital for treatment can be combined with the number of such patients still awaiting treatment to justify expansion of existing facilities or the construction of new ones. Birth, death, and migration rates may be used to predict the future size and composition of a regional population, and plans can be adapted accordingly to provide for a growing or shrinking demand for health care facilities. Income from taxes, bills, and contributions can similarly be predicted in order to estimate the financial burden on the community for additional facilities. Finally, the person or family receiving services from the consortium of health care professionals supplies information on the provision of health care. These figures are collated with others to provide a statistical picture of the operation of the hospital or health care system. Unthinking use of such figures can lead to statements such as those which have appeared in many newspapers and magazines, namely, that comprehensive health plans reduce all health costs by 50%. Later we shall study how to evaluate such statements.

All the above uses of objective data are directly related to the treatment of the patient or his family, and these uses justify the generation of this data. However, as a bonus, the information generated for operational uses may serve as a basis for the study of the system itself—whether it be the work load and work practices of an individual physician or dentist, the effectiveness of social policies such as Medicare, or changes in laws regarding abortion.

The numerical information collected in a hospital is invaluable to the hospital administrator in describing the operation of that hospital. He would, however, be inundated by trivia if he had no way of reducing all this information to its essential features. Alternatively he may select only that information that is inconsistent with previous data to indicate areas where the system is "going out of control" or to isolate an area where a problem is likely to arise. This practice has been called **exception reporting**.

The scientific method evolved in the laboratory, where the scientist could manipulate his material or his system. Problems in health care, however, are not soluble by such means (or they would already have been solved). For ethical and logistic reasons manipulation of a health care system is not generally possible. Nevertheless, many different systems can be offered to the public and those that survive and grow are, in general, best adapted to serve the needs of that community. There is, therefore, ample opportunity to study the workings of different health care systems in this country. This book seeks to prepare the reader to use wisely the information generated from such systems.

1.5 ANALYSIS OF HEALTH CARE INFORMATION

A supervisor can easily be overwhelmed by the welter of information produced by the health care system in his charge. Major Greenwood, in a discussion of a paper by Yule (1934), states that "the statistical method has been introduced precisely because the power of the human mind to grasp a number of particulars is limited." Thus, it is unreasonable to expect a medical superintendent to know the names and details of all the patients in his charge at a given point in time. He will typically remember such facts as that about 30% of the hospital's patients are children and that the number of new patients admitted ranges from 3 to 15 daily. Statistical principles are therefore concerned with the reduction of data to its basic constituents so that this information may be more easily understood and used. However, the basic (raw) data should not be discarded without careful thought, because it may be needed to answer a question arising about an individual patient or to check the original arithmetic (fiscal audits) that produced the summary statistics. In addition, research workers may want to analyze the basic data from quite different points of view to examine the workings of the system or to examine epidemiological theories on etiology and associations of diseases, etc. Today it is possible to store basic information systematically, accurately, and cheaply on computer tapes. The use of the computer in the management of health care information is described more fully in Chapter 12.

The value of the reduction of information depends on how representative the resultant statistics are of the population in which we are interested. (Remember this might be an artificial population of numbers.) If the information comes from a complete census (in which all the items in the population are measured), then the only point we can raise is the relevance of the measure to the problem at hand. For example, if it had been shown in a census of participants enrolled in a comprehensive health care plan that there was a 50% reduction in hospitalization compared with similar national standards, then one might ask whether this is relevant. The reduction may have occurred by the plan's physicians treating members in their offices or in the patients' homes. A more relevant question would be, "Do health plan members enjoy better health at less cost than others who are comparable?" With sample data (in which not all items in the population of interest are measured) we can also question the relevancy of the information gathered. In addition we must concern ourselves with the validity of generalizing our information from the sample to the population of interest. Thus a National Health Center Household Interview Study (Kelly, 1965), on the basis of 6672 sample adults, claims that 50% of the adult population of the United States have gingivitis and 25% destructive periodontal disease. The accuracy of the extrapolation from the sample to the total adult population of the United States depends on the representativeness of the individuals examined, as well as any variation in the standards used in deciding when a person has gingivitis or periodontal disease.

Errors in extrapolating from the sample to the population can arise in a number of ways. The first is representativeness. If the method of selecting samples is such that unrepresentative samples are obtained, these samples will give **biased** estimates. For example, if the above researchers deliberately selected individuals who had not visited a dentist in the past year, then the result would be biased and high. If, however, the individuals were sampled or selected from lists of people who had just had routine dental examinations, then the estimate would be biased and low. Another source of error is caused by sampling. There is no guarantee (indeed it is most unlikely) that if a second sample were selected it would give the same estimate as the first. Generally, we attempt to prevent bias by selecting samples and statistics that give unbiased estimates and then calculate the **accuracy** of the estimate from such samples to give confidence limits (Chapter 7) for the value in the population. Other problems, however, arise in such predictions, such as how to handle nonresponders and people who move away or die.

Finally, we reach the two least accurate forms of information on which to estimate a population value. These are the single fact and the subjective impression. The single fact may, of course, be considered a sample of size one. However, it is more likely to be selected to prove a point. The quoted single fact may not be verifiable, in that it may have been misreported, reported out of context, or even invented. Impressions are also suspect in that they usually conform to the general attitude of the person holding them and involve subjective judgments or criteria not generally acceptable. This is not to imply that objective information is always reliable. Daryll Huff's *How to Lie with Statistics* points out the traps laid by the unscrupulous for the unwary (Huff, 1954).

1.6 SUMMARY

The art of using statistics effectively consists of knowing how far one can safely generalize from available information. This requires an intimate knowledge of the system so that irrelevant differences can be ignored and important factors taken into account. We grow accustomed to regularity in nature and in our own social structures. Thus, skin sections taken from different individuals will contain cells identical in their composition, structure, and functioning in spite of the fact that the donors may differ by sex, age, and color. However, if we examine these specimens in more detail, we discover the polar bodies that differentiate somatic cells by sex and, theoretically, we should be able to distinguish cells from members of different races and cells from donors of different ages. The point here is that at a certain level or in certain essential ways all human body cells seem to be alike but more detailed examination shows them to differ.

Health care is similarly based on the fact that to a certain degree people and their diseases are alike, in spite of individual differences in tolerance to drugs and of incompatibilities in blood transfusion. Doctors, dentists, group practices, hospitals, and health districts are all both similar to and different from others in their class. By and large, the closer together in space and time, the more similar are patients' diseases, professional practices, hospital procedures, and personnel training. Time can result in things growing apart (identical twins, two newly founded hospitals) or in their growing together (husband's and wife's attitudes, legal pressures for uniformity of standards). These then are some of the influences on and considerations in the use of health care information. In the following chapters, these points are elaborated and extended. It is, however, important for the reader to have some feeling for the total framework in which the following isolated topics appear. In practice, they are not separate.

LITERATURE CITED

Huff, D. 1954. How to Lie with Statistics. W. W. Norton & Company Inc., New York.

Kelly, J. E. 1965. Periodontal Disease in Adults. United States 1960—62. NCHS Ser. 11, No. 12, U.S. Government Printing Office, Washington.

Yule, G. U. 1934. On some points relating to the vital statistics of occupational mortality. J. Roy. Statistic. Soc., Ser. A, 97:1.

FURTHER READING

Acheson, E. D. 1967. Medical Record Linkage. Published for Nuffield Trust by the Oxford Univ. Press, London.

Quade, E. S. 1970. On the Limitations of Quantitative Analysis. Paper 4530. Rand Corporation, Santa Monica, Calif.

2

Collection, Presentation, and Interpretation of Health Care Information

2.1 COLLECTION

2.1.1 Measurements and Classifications

The purpose for which information is to be gathered must be clearly stated and understood. This objective determines what measurements or questions are used and which items or people will be the source of the information. The items to be measured or the information to be gathered must be unambiguously defined. Thus, when we talk of the United States does this include its territories or not? Does the United States' population include citizens in the armed forces who are abroad or not? Does the term "physician" refer to M.D.'s only or does it include osteopaths? What about part-time and retired physicians? Do hospital beds include cribs? Do hospital admissions include patients discharged on the day of admission? Do births include stillbirths? Are multiple births counted as one or many? The population of interest consists of all those items or informants who might possibly yield information. From this population or **frame**, the items actually to be measured are selected according to well-defined and clearly stated sampling rules. Thus, weight gains in the first two months of life and 30 albino Wistar rats fed on a

11

restricted diet are measurements referrable to all newborn rats of that strain (assuming the homogeneity of the strain).

It is convenient to describe the collection and treatment of data by the type of data collected. Basically these are measurements and classification. A **measurement** has an underlying unit that may be measured in fractions. A measurement is therefore potentially continuous and can in many cases be both positive and negative. Weight gain is a measurement in that it has an underlying unit (grams or pounds). We can therefore get values to arbitrarily small fractions of a gram or pound (depending on the sensitivity of our scales) and we can conceive of a negative weight gain or weight loss. A **classification** on the other hand consists of the number of different states that a unit can have. Thus, the human ABO blood group system has four recognizable types (A, B, AB, and O) and we can classify each person's blood as belonging to one and only one of these. There is no underlying unit since human blood is classified according to its reactivity in certain tests. Note that each category of a classification is mutually exclusive (a person's blood belongs to only one of these four exclusive categories). Note also that the classification is exhaustive (a person's blood must fall in one or another of these categories). In addition, a classification is more subjective than a measurement. The ordering of the categories is generally arbitrary (the ordering of the form ABO blood types comes from the alphabet, which is itself arbitrary) and the number of categories may be variable (a serologist may discriminate between type A_1 and type A_2 blood and use the classification ($A_1 : A_2 : B : A_1B : A_2B : O$), whereas another investigator may simply be interested in the proportion with gene A in their blood type and use the classification (A and other) where A is composed of types A and AB). The form of classification used is therefore decided upon by the collector of the information as is the minimum fraction of a unit to be used in a measurement. Some classifications have an implicit ordering of the categories of which they are composed. These classifications are sometimes considered to be measurements and are used as though they were. They lack an underlying unit, however. Thus, the classification of health as (dead : severely ill : moderately ill : slightly ill : recovering : well) clearly has no underlying unit, nor do many other psychological or sociological scales. A **count** is a limiting form of a classification with only one category. The number of children in a family is a count and not a measurement since fractions of a child are impossible. The concept of the average number of children in a family as, say, 2.2 demonstrates how frequently counts are treated as measurements. It is illogical to treat a count as a measurement but it is often convenient to do so.

2.1.2 Errors Arising in the Collection of Information

Systematic errors may be introduced in making measurements by parallax or by other biases of the investigator. Occasionally measurements have to be made indirectly, such as estimating the volume of the skull from intercristal measurements of the head. In such indirect measurements there are two possible sources of error: the original readings and the method of estimation. In the first instance, small errors in the basic readings may be inflated when combined in a formula to give an estimate of some variable that cannot be measured directly. Therefore, some of the basic readings may be more important than others and more care must be taken to reduce errors from these sources. In the second case, the formula used to convert basic readings into an indirect estimate may be inaccurate.

Information gathered by questionnaires distributed among individual patients, clients, or participants in a health scheme is subject to other errors. The respondent may answer a different question from the one asked. This lack of communication may not be obvious to the pollster. The questions themselves may be biased or the respondent may give the answer that he thinks is expected or desired. Finally, the accuracy of a reply will be affected by the respondent's memory and his desire to cooperate. Special problems arise in interviewing children, the sick, aged, institutionalized, and mentally infirm. The problem of how to handle nonrespondents, people who have died or moved out of the area, also arises. Generally, the population is defined as consisting of only living residents of the area, thus avoiding the latter problem. Those who do not respond are approached several times before being considered nonrespondents. The effect of nonrespondents on a survey can be calculated by assuming first that they all answered a given question negatively, then that they all answered that question positively, and finally that their answers were proportional to those of the respondents. These calculations give upper and lower limits of the nonsampling error due to nonresponse. The accuracy of the respondent's questions may be checked by asking the same question, phrased differently, several times or by correlating a respondent's replies with other sources of information. However, there is no absolutely certain method of validating all the information gathered. Respondents may give misinformation deliberately or they may give incorrect information unconsciously. Few surveys ever received a complete response from all of the members of the sample and few samples are entirely representative of the population of interest. However, errors tend to cancel each other and the results of one survey are judged by their degree of consistency with similar surveys and with other knowledge, so the situation is not hopeless.

Records should be kept in permanent books or on approved specially designed forms. The name of the investigation and of the investigator, the date the information was collected, and the identification of the item measured should all be recorded. A standard number of decimal places should be decided upon for each separate measurement and numerical data should be recorded in a straightforward manner to allow for easy reading. Thus, the use of the pen is advocated rather than pencil. Decimal points should be aligned. Changes may be made by drawing a line through the number to be changed and writing the correct number above it.

There should be ample space on forms for the size of the typical entry, and provision should be made for continuation sheets. Classifications should refer to a single variable and should not be a combination of several, i.e., rather than (A♂ : A♀ : B♂ : B♀ : AB♂ : AB♀ : O♂ : O♀) the separate classifications (A : B : AB : O) and (♂ : ♀) are preferred. In making a complex investigation it is sometimes beneficial to describe the recording procedures by the use of a **flow chart** (Figure 2.1) specifying how various eventualities should be handled. Also, it is useful to perform a **pilot** survey, which can be used to evaluate the accuracy of the questions and the record forms to be used in the investigation.

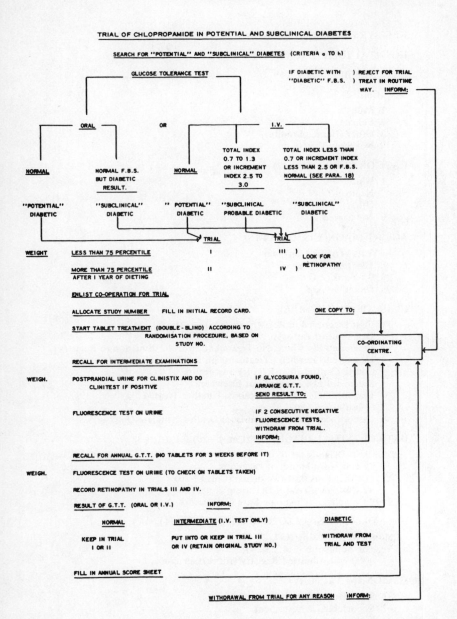

Figure 2.1. Sample flow chart for trial of a new drug. (From the British Diabetic Society collaborative study of Cholorpropramide.)

REGISTRY NUMBER (Col. 1-2)

HOSPITAL IDENTIFICATION (Col. 3-5)

CASE NUMBER (Col. 6-11)

SEX (Col. 12)

   1 Male
   2 Female
   3 Other (Hermaphrodite)
   9 Not Stated

RACE OR COLOR (Col. 13)

   1 White
   2 Negro
   3 Other
   9 Not Stated

AGE AT DIAGNOSIS (Col. 14-15)

   In Years as of Last Birthday
   00 Less than One Year
   98 98 Years or Older
   99 Unknown Age

CLASS OF CASE (Col. 16)

   1 First Diagnosed in Registry Hospital or Clinic
   2 Diagnosed at Autopsy
   3 Diagnosed Elsewhere, No Treatment Prior to Admission to Registry
   4 Diagnosed Elsewhere, Treatment Initiated Elsewhere and Same
      Course Continued at Registry Institution
   5 Diagnosed Elsewhere, Treat Elsewhere
   6 Diagnosed Elsewhere, Unknown Whether Treated
   7 Consultation Only
   8 Case Information Obtained from Death Certificate Only

DATE OF INITIAL DIAGNOSIS (Col. 17-20)

   Month of Diagnosis (Col. 17-18)
      99 Unknown Month of Diagnosis
   Year of Diagnosis (last two digits) (Col. 19-20)
      99 Unknown Year of Diagnosis
   9999 Completely Unknown Date of Diagnosis

DATE OF ADMISSION TO REGISTRY (Col. 21-24)

   Month of Admission (Col. 21-22)
   Year of Admission (Col. 23-24)
      0000 Not Admitted Registry (for certain cases)

MALIGNANCY (Col. 25)

   1 Specified as Malignant
   2 Reportable by Agreement
   3 Followed for Special Interest

Continued

Figure 2.2. Extract from a typical coding form for a cancer tumor registry.

PRIMARY SITE (Col. 26-28)

Code Based on International Classification of Diseases,
1955 Revision, WHO—with the following modifications:

For ISC 191.8 and 190.8, the 0.8 designates more than one
lesion regardless of location.

ISC 204.0: Acute, chronic, or unspecified lymphatic leukemia.
ISC 204.1: Acute, chronic, or unspecified myeloid leukemia.
ISC 204.1: Acute, chronic, or unspecified monocytic leukemia.
ISC 204.3: Acute leukemia unspecified as to type.

Polycythemia vera is coded to ISC 204.4

For cases Reportable by Agreement or followed for Special
Interest (2 or 3 in Field J) the code in Field K is the code
number that would have been assigned had the neoplasm been considered
malignant.

SEQUENCE NUMBER (Col. 29)

0 One Primary Only
1 First of Two or More Primaries
2 Second of Two or More Primaries
3 Third or Later Primary
9 Unspecified Sequence Number

HISTOLOGICAL TYPE (Col. 30-32)

Code per Manual of Tumor Nomenclature and Coding American
Cancer Society, 1951, with the following additions:

X10   Negative Pathology
X20   No Histology
XOX   Pathology Data Not Coded; Not Being Submitted

For multiple skin cancer summary cards, use the following
code numbers:

15.6 All Squamous Cell Carcinomas
15.7 All Basal Cell Carcinomas
15.8 More than one histological type represented by the
        individual lesions
15.9 At least one unspecified histological type—but only
        if not already classificable as 15.8.

DIAGNOSTIC CONFIRMATION (Col. 33)

1 Positive Histology
2 Positive Exfoliative Cytology, No Information Concerning Histology
3 Positive Exfoliative Cytology and Negative Histology
4 Positive Microscope Confirmation, Method Not Specified
5 Not Microscopically Confirmed
9 Unspecified Whether or Not Microscopically Confirmed

Figure 2.2. *Continued.*

This validation should include a trial of the coding forms to be used if the data, especially in large-scale studies, are to be analyzed by a computer. Figure 2.2 is an example of the detail necessary in such coding forms. It describes the coding used in a cancer tumor registry.

2.2 PRESENTATION

2.2.1 Numerical Conventions

The number of decimal places in an observation should indicate the precision of the measurement. For example, blood pressure is measured to the nearest mm Hg. However, if one reads that a systolic blood pressure is 123.2, one can assume that the person who recorded the blood pressure used a sensitive manometer which could be read in tenths of a mm Hg.

It is generally assumed that, when repeated observations are made, the person making these observations measures with the same degree of accuracy each time. The same number of decimal points should therefore be used throughout. Thus, if one were describing the elevation of systolic blood pressure, where this is calculated as "after treatment minus before treatment," one might measure to one decimal, e.g., 0.4 mm Hg. In this case one would expect that a zero reading be given as 0.0. This would mean that no detectable difference was observed to the nearest tenth of a mm Hg. An anomaly arises when measurements containing fractions are converted into decimal notations. Thus, if body weight were measured to the nearest quarter pound, because the quarter pound was the smallest division on the scale, one might record a weight of 170¼ as 170.25 lb. This figure, however, suggests that the weight was measured to the nearest hundredth of a pound, which would not be the case. There is no easy solution to this anomaly except to work in the most basic units available, in this case quarter pounds. Thus, decimals are eliminated: 170¼ would then be recorded as 681 quarter pounds.

Another useful convention in the presentation of numerical data is the expression of comparative statistics in relation to a single base. Authors sometimes use a combination of **odds**, fractions, and percentages. The following extract provides an example: "From an earlier paper we showed that the odds of having another affected child were 1/13. In this study the proportion of affected children (excluding the propositus) was 8/57." The difficulty of comparing 1 in 13 with 8 in 57 can be alleviated by writing, "From an earlier paper we showed that the proportion of women having another affected child was 0.1 or 1/14. In this study the proportion of affected children (excluding the propositus) was 0.14 or 8/57." It is now clear that the current study reveals a slightly higher frequency of affected children than the older study did, but that this information is unreliable because of the small number of cases on which the first estimate was based. This is revealed by its expression to only one decimal point. Again, "The pH of sweat in 11 of the normal sibs was measured, and this was found to be elevated in 5 (45.45%)," might better be written as, "The pH of sweat in all of the normal sibs was measured and this was found to be elevated in about 0.5 (5/11)." The expression of all numerical data in terms of a percentage leads to a spurious degree of sensitivity if the base is much less than a hundred. Percentages are often grossly misleading especially when no total number of items used is supplied. Consider the statement "In the current study 43% of patients with regional ileitis had blood group O. This was lower than the 56% reported in our earlier study." This implies that regional ileitis is changing in its relationship to blood group O. However, when one realizes that 43% consists of 3 patients having blood group O out of a total of 7 and the 56% consists of 5 out of 9 patients, the difference in the percentages immediately loses importance.

2.2.2 Condensation of Information in One Variable

The reader is seldom presented with raw data. Exceptions to this are certain scientific journals that print the original information on which an article is written because this may lead to further research based on the published data. Thus, in human genetics, family pedigrees and detailed information about each family are published and tabulated, even though the authors are interested only in presenting an overall mutation rate. Occasionally the

Table 2.1. Frequency distribution of 320 newborn infants in parity

Parity	1	2	3	4	5	6	7	8	>8	Total
Frequency	138	119	35	16	6	3	3	0	0	320
Percentage	43	37	11	5	2	1	1	0	0	100

original measurements are recorded so that the reader can deduce the range of variation in the variable. Inevitably, however, condensation of information is necessary as the number of observations increases.

A single measure (e.g., duration of labor) or a classification (e.g., parity of new born : first : second : etc.) can be summarized by a **frequency distribution**. In the case of a classification, the reader is given the number or frequency of items falling into a given category and, usually, the equivalent percentage. If 320 newborns had been classified according to parity (number of previous children born to that mother +1) we would have, not the 320 separate parity figures, but a table such as Table 2.1.

A large number of measurements of a single variable may be treated similarly by subdividing the measure into a number of intervals. Note that we are losing a certain amount of this measurement's precision by agreeing to treat it as though it were of classification. Thus, if associated with each of the 320 parities we had also the duration of the mother's labor recorded in hours and minutes, we could agree to measure only to the nearest hour to get Table 2.2.

Table 2.2. Frequency distribution of duration of labor (in hours) in 320 deliveries

Duration of labor	<1	1-2	2-3	3-4	4-5	5-6	6-7	7-8	>8	Total
Frequency	10	6	16	48	115	67	32	13	13	320
Percentage	3	2	5	15	36	21	10	4	4	100

In both these illustrations, the categories are mutually exclusive and exhaustive (1–2 hours' duration of labor means a labor lasting at least one hour and less than two hours). Note also that percentages are given for ease of comparison with other series in which the total number differs from 320.

Numerical or tabular presentations of information in one variable, such as those given in Tables 2.1, and 2.2, are called one-way **frequency tables.** Graphic presentations equivalent to these tables are the bar graph and histogram. **A bar graph** consists of a number of rectangular bars, where the length of each bar represents the frequency of a given category. Bar graphs are usually most effective for emphasizing differences in individual categories in a series of classifications. The bars in a bar graph should be of equal width and may be either vertical (Figure 2.3) or horizontal (Figure 2.4), although vertical bars are usually used to present data classified by time.

Bar graphs may also be used to compare two or more sets of data classified in the same way. This is done by placing bars side by side and using different markings to distinguish the sets of data, as shown in Figure 2.5. Other versions of the bar graph are the component parts graph, the pictograph, and the map graph. A **component parts graph** may be used to show relationships among

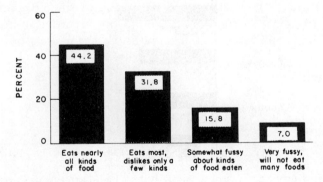

Figure 2.3. Percentage of children aged 6–11, by degree of selectivity with food, United States, 1963–65. (From *The Health of Children, 1970,* The National Center for Health Statistics, U.S. Department of Health, Education, and Welfare, Public Health Service Publication No. 2121, p. 46, chart 50.)

Figure 2.4. Infant mortality rates; selected countries in rank order. *Note:* This is not a frequency distribution. (From *The Health of Children, 1970,* The National Center for Health Statistics, U.S. Department of Health, Education, and Welfare, Public Health Service Publication No. 2121, p. 4, chart 1.)

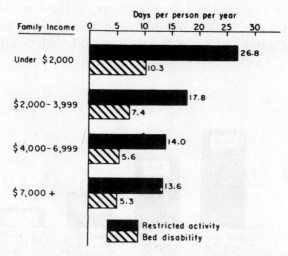

Figure 2.5. Number of restricted-activity and bed-disability days per person per year, by family income. (From *Disability Days, United States, July 1961–June 1962,* The National Center for Health Statistics, U.S. Department of Health, Education, and Welfare, Public Health Service Publication No. 1000, Ser. 10, No. 4, p. 9.)

22

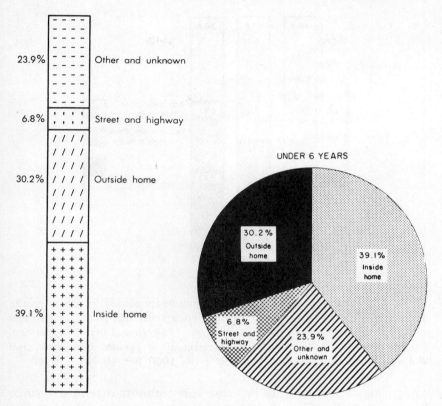

Figure 2.6. Percentage of injured children under 6 years of age by place of accident, United States, 1965–67. (Adapted from *The Health of Children, 1970,* The National Center for Health Statistics, U.S. Department of Health, Education, and Welfare, Public Health Service Publication No. 2121, p. 24, chart 24.)

Figure 2.7. Percentage of injured children under 6 years of age by place of accident, United States, 1965–67. (From *The Health of Children, 1970,* The National Center for Health Statistics, U.S. Department of Health, Education, and Welfare, Public Health Service Publication No. 2121, p. 24, chart 24.)

various individual parts of a whole. The relationships can be expressed as proportions, but more often they are expressed as percentages. The component parts are often shown as parts of a bar (Figure 2.6) or as segments of a circle or pie (Figure 2.7), with the bar or pie representing the whole and the segments the component parts. Component parts graphs can also be used for

Figure 2.8. Percentage distribution of impairments caused by injury in the home attributed to falls, by age. (From *Impairments Due to Injury by Class and Type of Accident, United States, July 1959–June 1961,* The National Center for Health Statistics, U.S. Department of Health, Education, and Welfare, Public Health Service Publication No. 1000, Ser. 10, No. 6, p. 4.)

comparing sets of data. In this case bars are more often used, since it is easier to compare segments of bars than segments of a circle. Figure 2.8 is an example of a component parts graph used to compare several sets of data. Figure 2.9 is a pictograph or picto-

Figure 2.9. Deaths per 100,000 policyholders of the Metropolitan Life Insurance Company from special diseases of the heart, February 1952. (From F. E. Croxton, *Elementary Statistics with Applications in Medicine and the Biological Sciences,* Dover Publications, New York, 1953, p. 38.)

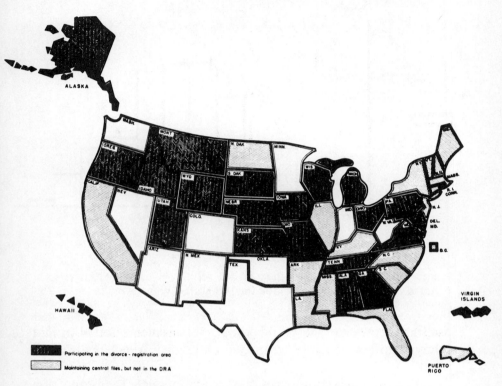

Figure 2.10. Divorce registration areas and other states maintaining central files of divorce and annulment records, 1965. (From *Divorce Statistics Analysis, United States, 1964 and 1965,* The National Center for Health Statistics, U.S. Department of Health, Education, and Welfare, Public Health Service Publication No. 1000, Ser. 21, No. 17, p. 52.)

gram. A **pictograph** uses picture symbols to represent data, where each symbol represents a fixed amount of data, and the number of symbols indicates the magnitude.

Another type of chart that can be used is a **statistical map** such as the one in Figure 2.10. Statistical maps present quantitative information by geographical location. The information is plotted on the geographical units being compared. In a frequency table the data for a single measure can be presented graphically as a **histogram**. A frequency histogram is shown in Figure 2.11. Usually the measure is marked off in intervals along the horizontal axis and the frequency is marked off along the vertical axis. The height of

Figure 2.11. Frequency histogram of cell volume in cubic centimeters per hundred cubic centimeters of blood for 100 normal young women.

each bar represents the frequency of measurements found in that interval. Either absolute frequency or **relative frequency** may be used.

Since the area above each class interval equals the proportion of observations within that interval, the histogram shows quickly how the data is distributed over the entire range of values. We can see that most of the data in Figure 2.11 are clustered about the center with fewer values at either extreme.

2.2.3 Condensation of Information in Two Variables

The three possible combinations of two variables by type are a measure by a measure, a measure by a classification, and a classification by a classification. The first of these, a measure by a measure, occurs whenever we have paired readings on a unit of the population and both these readings are measures. For example, in a study of people discharged from a hospital, we may have the amount of their bills and the duration of their stay or we may have the weekly amount of money each spent on food and the number of calories consumed each week for a given period of time. Such paired measurements can be plotted on a graph or a

Figure 2.12. Relationship of age and weight in children by sex and race. *Note:* Each child would be represented by a point in the graph, not necessarily falling on a line. The scatter of these individual plots about the appropriate line demonstrates the variation of individuals about the presumed age-weight relationship. (From *The Health of Children, 1970,* The National Center for Health Statistics, U.S. Department of Health, Education, and Welfare, Public Health Service Publication No. 2121, p. 39, chart 40.)

scatter diagram on which each pair of observations for a given unit is represented by a point on the graph. The object of making such a graph is to demonstrate or to find a relationship between the two continuous variables. Figure 2.12 is an example of such a graph.

When the variables are both classifications, one can present the data in the form of a two-way table in which one classification defines the rows and the other defines the columns of the table. Each cell of the table illustrates the number or frequency of items that have those two attributes defined by the row and column that intersect in the cell. (See Table 2.3.) The numbers in a two-way table such as Table 2.3 may be reduced to percentages in one of three ways. The frequency in a given cell may be expressed as a percentage of the row total, of the column total, or of the grand

Table 2.3. Occurrence of major salivary gland tumors

	Parotid	Submaxillary	Sublingual	Total
Benign	501	47	0	548
Malignant	231	54	3	288
Total	732	101	3	836

From: W.G. Shafer, M.K. Hine, and B.M. Levy, *Textbook of Oral Pathology*, 2nd ed., Saunders, Philadelphia, 1964, p. 181.

total. Thus, in Table 2.3, there are 231 malignant parotid tumors. Depending on our interest this number may be expressed as 31.6% (231/732)—which is the percentage of all parotid tumors which were malignant—or as 80.2% (231/288)—which is the percentage of all malignant tumors found in the parotid gland—or as 27.6% (231/836)—which is the percentage of all tumors that were both malignant and located in the parotid gland.

Since we can degrade a measure to an ordered classification (e.g., age to the nearest year or young : middle-aged : old), it is simple to present pairs of observations that include both a measurable variable and a classification. We treat the measurable variable as though it were a classification and present the data in a two-way table. In the example on salivary gland tumors (Table 2.3), we may wish to tabulate information relating the age of the patient to the type of tumor (benign, malignant). This would lead to a table in which age is treated like an ordered classification (young, middle-aged, old; or more precisely <35 yr, 35 to 60 yr, >60 yr). Note that the classification used to accommodate a measure in a two-way table is at the discretion of the writer and will usually reflect the known distribution of values of the measure. Thus, if the ages of all 836 patients in Table 2.3 were between 35 and 60 yr, the table would be relatively uninformative since two of the three age categories would be empty. Usually tables that contain many empty cells should be omitted or reconstructed. However, the opposite tendency, that of presenting tables or graphs that contain too much information, should be avoided also, since these are often too difficult to read. It is sometimes possible to present data on a

Figure 2.13. Cost of installation and operation of elevators of different sizes. (From *Problems and Progress in Medical Care,* Second Series, Ed. G. McLachlan. Published for the Nuffield Provincial Hospitals Trust by Oxford University Press, 1966, p. 194, Figure 4.)

classification and a measurement by assuming that the classification is a measure. This is only possible where the classification is ordered (underweight, normal, overweight) and is only recommended where the ordered classification is a count (size of family), for then there is a unit (although not a divisible unit). Figure 2.13 is an example of this type of graph.

2.2.4 Statistical Condensation for More than Two Variables

In most health-related surveys, many variables are obtained for each item in the population. The limitation of the printed page to two dimensions restricts the publication of many multidimensional tables. These tables are usually printed for the two variables of interests at a specified level or levels of the other associated variables. Thus, the birth rate per 1000 women may be published by age of mother (in 5-yr age groups, say), by race, by region, and by socioeconomic status. This information could be presented in any one of six different ways, tabulating the birth rate by 1) age and race, 2) age and region, 3) age and status, 4) race and region, 5) race and status, or 6) region and status. In each presentation, tables would be given for the two chosen variables at different levels of the other two variables.

* This assessment must be regarded as relative and in no sense absolute.

Figure 2.14. Nomogram for assessing seminal quality from spermatozoan number, motility number, and head normality. A straight line is drawn between the observed spermatozoal number (on scale I) and the observed percentage of motile spermatozoa (on scale III). The intersection of this line with scale II is now connected by another straight line with the observed percentage of normal head forms on scale V. The intersection of this line with scale IV gives the fertility index. (From E. W. Page and F. Houlding, *Fertil. Steril.*, 2:140 (1951).)

Statistical tables used are generally multidimensional. Thus, we may want the value of a statistic associated with a given probability and with several other values, such as degrees of freedom and parameter values. One of the difficulties in using appropriate statistical tests is using the table to find the probability associated with that test or the sample size required.

Nomograms attempt to simplify the use of complicated tables. A **nomogram** is a graphic aid in displaying the relationships implicit in a table. Generally, a nomogram consists of a small number of lines or curves with variable scales. A straight line joining values on two of these scales cuts another scale at a point that is then read. This value is the required answer. In some cases the nomogram has more than three lines. This happens in the determination of male fertility when the procedure must be repeated. Thus, in the nomogram given in Figure 2.14, a line joining values of sperm count and percentage of sperm still motile two hours after ejaculation gives a value on an intermediate scale. A second straight line is then drawn between this value and the percentage of normal head forms to determine the value on the fertility index. A second case of a nomogram with more than three lines is the combination of two different nomograms into one. For example, in estimating upper and lower **confidence limits** the separate nomograms for the upper and lower confidence limits are combined (see Dixon and Massey, 1957, Table A-9). Conversion from one scale to another (e.g., from degrees Fahrenheit to degrees Centigrade) can be achieved by a degraded nomogram with only one line labeled on both sides with the two scales. Nomograms are easy to use but may not intrinsically be precise for certain combinations of values. Also, errors may be made in drawing the line and reading the value. In addition, a nomogram cannot yield the number of significant digits of a table because of the difficulties of reading a nonlinear scale that is perhaps very condensed. However, this device is extremely valuable for those applications in which one wants to find the answer quickly (e.g., whether a patient is overweight in terms of his height and weight, whether a hospital's income is consistent with its number of beds and number of employees).

2.2.5 Statistical Summaries of Health Care Information

In the above sections we have been concerned with the tabular and graphic presentation of data. We can, of course, reduct this information still further by giving only certain summary or descriptive statistics. These are measures of location (averages), measures of dispersion (range and standard deviations), and measures of association (χ^2 and correlation). Many other statistics have been invented to summarize data but these are sufficient to illustrate the procedure. Note, however, that the number of items examined should always be given. It is misleading to report that 33% of births in a hospital are illegitimate without reporting the number on which this percentage is based. It could mean simply that three mothers were delivered and that one of them was not married. The same requirement holds in the presentation of measurable information. For example, consider the information that the average time a hospital keeps mothers in bed after childbirth is 2 days, 3 hours, and 41 minutes. This is misleading if the average is based on a small number of mothers and the reader is not told what the number is. In examples like the above, a large number of decimal places may be used but the result is an erroneous impression of great precision.

Tables and graphs often use summary statistics instead of frequencies. This is a convenient way of "boiling down" a long list of observations with many variables of which at least one is a measure. Thus, the information on weight by age, sex, and race in Figure 2.12 could be presented by showing the average weight in each age, sex, and race group. In Figure 3.1 the "average" number of work days lost is reported for each of several different occupational groups. A comparison of two "averages" for each family income group is shown in Figure 2.5 in the form of a bar graph. A statistical graph such as the one in Figure 2.15 may show a summary statistic rather than the classification of each state as belonging to one of a number of different classes, as in Figure 2.10. Pseudo-statistics may also be given in tabular or graphic form. Thus, Figure 2.4 shows the infant mortality rate (deaths per 1000 live births) in each of several countries.

In order to understand properly the information contained in

Figure 2.15. Provisional estimates of days of bed disability per person per year. (From *Synthetic State Estimates of Disability*, The National Center for Health Statistics, U.S. Department of Health, Education, and Welfare, U.S. Public Health Service Publication No. 1759, p. 7.)

a table or graph, one should be able to visualize the basic data. What units were examined? What variables were observed on these units? How was the list reduced? Are the entries in the table frequencies or summary statistics?

2.3 INTERPRETATION

The following chapters present the necessary background for a proper understanding of the interpretation of statistical information. Points raised in this section are therefore covered in detail later.

There is a tendency to accept a claim made in a published paper either because of the author's reputation or because of the reputation of the journal. Sometimes a claim is rejected because it is not in accord with current theories. Thus, many people do not accept the validity of claims supporting the existence of ESP (extrasensory perception) because to do so would challenge our general view of the physical world. The validity of a claim is also dependent on the validity of the study from which the claim was generated. To accept that a given conclusion can logically be drawn from the available information requires a knowledge of statistical principles and of the design of investigations. (See Chapter 13.)

If editors, accreditation boards, and other review bodies did not exist, we would be entitled to doubt the existence of any system generating the data presented to us. A printed statement to the effect that the minimum wage for a given health professional is $6.50 per hour does not make that wage a reality. Recourse to the basic data should always be given to qualified people and bona fide investigators. If one concludes that the information is valid, one must ask whether it has been properly analyzed. Arithmetical errors can occur in the calculation of an average. A more serious problem will arise if the person manipulating the data used an incorrect procedure or misnamed the result. Frequently, in the hands of the nonstatisticians "the standard deviation" is incorrectly substituted for "the standard error." The possibility of these kinds of errors requires that, where possible, the raw data be made available for re-examination.

One must ask whether a given question is relevant to the study. Irrelevant information may be supplied to impress the reader with the completeness of the study. This information is likely to be unimportant. However, it may answer someone's questions about comparability of the study population with the general population. More serious is the situation in which the question asked or the measure made is not in accord with the original formulation of the study objectives. Thus, in a study of oral hygiene one cannot assume that the cleanliness of the teeth is a measure of the frequency of cleaning by toothbrush. Some teeth may be clean because of diet, e.g., more fruit may be eaten by one group than by another. Conversely, a person whose teeth show calcification may be brushing his teeth but he may be predisposed to calcification, may have poor mastication, or a poor diet.

In most applications, the information is collated for only a fraction of all the items in the population of interest. Thus, in a study of dental amalgams, the deterioration of conservative fillings may be examined only in the premolar teeth. A study of the number of years nurses must spend on full-time education before they are qualified may include the years spent by nurses from each of the 50 states but may be limited to include only one school in each state. Similarly a study of the demand for comprehensive health care may be based on a random sample of heads of households in one region that is covered by a health maintenance organization (HMO). There are various ways of justifying the representativeness of a population sample from which one wishes to make inferences. One way is simply to assert that the sample is representative. In doing so, we are saying that the sampled items are fundamentally no different from the items not sampled (with regard to the variable measured). Thus, a dentist might assert that an amalgam with good resistance to deterioration in premolar conservative fillings will also be a good amalgam in other types of fillings in other teeth. Since, however, different dentists might make different assertions there will probably be no censensus on the relative merits of a given amalgam. To validate the representativeness of a sample, we can compare the characteristics of the sample against known characteristics of the total population. Thus, in a survey of nurses' training, we might be able to compare the ages of the sampled nurses with those of all nurses. We may continue to do this for all variables known in both the sample and the population. If the distributions between sample and population agree, we have at least indirect support that the sample is representative of the population in respect to the variable of interest. However, this does not follow logically. For example, in an attitudinal survey of doctors' reasons for preferring group practice to individual practice, only 50% of the sample replied to the questionnaire. The investigators showed that the age and length of time since qualification of the respondents were similar to those of all registered practitioners in group practice. However, it cannot be assumed that the attitudes of the 50% who replied are representative of the attitudes of all doctors in group practice since their attitudes toward group practice may have affected the decision to reply.

Experts in sampling maintain that the only way to get a representative sample is to take a strictly **random sample**. While random sampling does not guarantee representativeness, there is little likelihood that a strictly random sample is seriously nonrepresentative. Statistical theory puts bounds on what the errors caused by random sampling variation will be. Thus, of the three situations mentioned above, the random sample of heads of households appears to provide the most representative sample. If a sample other than a random sample is to be considered representative, it is imperative that the person drawing conclusions from the sample data have an intimate knowledge of the system under study.

Instead of asking the survey expert or statistician, "How should I take my sample?" the layman usually asks, "How large should my sample be?" From the above it is clear that because of the biases involved, a small representative sample may be more valuable in supplying information about the population than a large unrepresentative sample. Nevertheless, having agreed, at least in theory, that sample items should be selected randomly from the population, the next task is to decide how many of these to take. As will be shown, the question can be answered once the desired accuracy of the estimate is specified. The small selected sample still can play a role—usually that of disproving a global statement.

Thus, the assertion that man's autosomal (nonreproductive) cells contained 48 chromosomes was disproved by Ford, Jacobs, and Lajtha (1958) who published the distribution of chromosome numbers in a relatively small number of skin cells. Similarly, the iatrogenic effects of thalidomide were established when it was demonstrated that the only factor common to those pregnancies producing this type of deformed child was that the mothers had taken thalidomide.

Mainland (1964) also gives the example of a dentist who examined 36,196 teeth for caries and reported his findings in terms of percentage of carious teeth. Clearly his report should have been in terms of the 1,870 children he examined since all the teeth in any one mouth are not **independent**. In an epidemiological study of an infectious disease one must allow for the clustering of individuals in families. For some infections, if one member of the family is infected, all members are likely to be infected at some time. Another example of clustering occurs in the evaluation of group therapy in psychiatric care. In this case it is the group of patients, not the individual patient, who may or may not respond to therapy. In other words, in any situation in which the measurements used might not be independent of other measurements, serious consideration should be given to the effect of this nonindependence and the sample should be redefined as clusters of measurements. Often, clustering has important implications for medical research scientists, who repeat their experiments on the same subjects or biological material, and who would be well advised to replicate the experiment using different subjects. The approach may be informative, especially if the investigator wishes to generalize his findings. Thus, the knowledge of the proportion of 80 subjects who faint after receiving an injection of distilled water is a different kind of information from that gained in a study in which one individual is given a series of 80 injections and the number of times he faints after injection is recorded.

In summary, then, before generalizing from sample results to the population of interest, we should check that the data exist, that the definitions, calculations, and methods used are correct, that the information gathered is relevant to the questions asked, and that the sample was selected randomly or that it is reasonable to assume that it is representative. Assumptions may have been made, often without being stated, in the statistical treatment of the data. These may be distributional (e.g., that the variable follows a **normal distribution**), or may be related to the independence of successive results, or to the equality of the variation in various different subgroups of a population. As indicated, the detection of arithmetical errors in a statistical report (such as calculating the ratio of two averages where the authors should have calculated the average ratio) or of inconsistencies (such as reporting the sample size differently in different sections of the report) throws suspicion on the quality of the report and makes the reader unwilling to accept the conclusions because of the possible existence of other errors that he cannot detect.

EXERCISES

(Note: For the locations of the figures and tables see the Lists of Figures and Tables on pp. ix and xi.)

2.1   Are the following variables measurements or classifications?
Duration of labor (Table 2.2)
Degree of selectivity with food (Figure 2.3)
Place of accident (Figure 2.6)
Type of accident (Figure 2.8)
Cause of death (Figure 2.9)
Divorce registration areas (Figure 2.10)
Age, weight, sex, race (Figure 2.12)
Type of gland (parotid, submaxillary, sublingual)
Type of tumor (benign, malignant) (Table 2.3)
Cost of installation (Figure 2.13)

2.2   Which of the following classifications are counts?
Parity (Table 2.1)
Elevator capacity, in persons (Figure 2.13)
Sequence number (Figure 2.2, Column 29)
Number of days sick
Average number of sick days per person per year (Figure 3.1)
Organ weight as percentage of total body weight (Figure 2.16)

2.3   a) Form one-way frequency tables from the graphs and histograms shown in Figures 2.3, 2.4, 2.6, 2.9, 2.10 and 2.11.
b) Form two-way frequency tables from Figures 2.5 and 2.8.
c) Draw histograms corresponding to Table 2.1, Figures 2.4, and 2.10.

Figure 2.16. Percentages of total body weight formed by various parts in the newborn human. (From F. E. Croxton, *Elementary Statistics with Applications in Medicine and the Biological Sciences,* Dover Publications, New York, 1953, p. 34.)

2.4 From the information presented in Tables 2.4 and 2.5 show how to calculate the absolute frequencies in each cell of Table 2.4. Why can we not use the same approach to calculate the absolute frequencies of residents and full-time employees in each cell of Table 2.4?

2.5 a) Given a three-way table formed from three variables, each of which is subdivided into three classes, how many cells does the table have?

b) A three-way table is formed from three variables, one of which contains 2 classes, one 4 classes, and one 5 classes. How many cells does the table have?

2.6 In correspondence with the director of a hospital in England, a research worker learns that the hospital contains between 200 and 250 beds and that these are arranged in 12 open-plan wards, each containing the same number of beds. From this information, deduce the possible range of values for the number of hospital beds per ward in this hospital.

2.7 How might Table 2.3 be converted to a single one-way frequency table? Form an additional seven one-way tables from Table 2.3. How many of these would you need to deduce the others?

Table 2.4. Percentage distribution of inpatient health facilities by type and bed size, 1967

Type of facility	Total facilities	<25 beds	25-49 beds	50-74 beds	75-90 beds	100-199 beds	200-299 beds	300-499 beds	500-999 beds	1,000 beds or more
All facilities	100.00	40.0	22.7	12.9	6.8	9.8	3.2	2.4	1.1	1.2
Short-stay hospitals	100.0	12.1	24.6	14.7	9.5	18.8	9.2	7.7	2.7	0.6
General	100.0	11.0	24.8	14.8	9.5	19.0	9.4	8.0	2.9	0.6
Specialty	100.0	32.9	20.5	13.6	10.0	14.8	4.8	1.8	0.3	1.2
Long-stay hospitals	100.0	6.6	14.0	12.4	9.6	16.4	7.7	7.3	8.0	18.0
General	100.0	4.0	10.2	7.9	5.6	13.6	10.2	15.8	14.7	18.1
Psychiatric	100.0	7.8	9.5	6.6	4.9	10.8	5.5	5.1	9.3	40.6
Geriatric and chronic	100.0	6.8	16.9	14.0	16.0	23.5	9.1	5.5	5.5	2.6
Tuberculosis	100.0	1.2	10.8	14.5	14.5	24.1	13.3	12.0	8.4	1.2
Other	100.0	10.3	27.0	27.0	10.8	14.6	3.8	3.8	1.6	1.1
Nursing care and related homes	100.0	44.5	25.4	14.1	6.7	7.5	1.1	0.5	0.1	0.0
Nursing care	100.0	25.1	32.8	20.2	10.0	10.1	1.2	0.5	0.1	0.0
Personal care with nursing care	100.0	48.6	22.8	11.4	5.2	8.7	2.1	1.0	0.2	0.1
Personal care without nursing care	100.0	85.4	10.8	2.5	0.5	0.8	0.1	--	--	--
Domiciliary care	100.0	85.5	9.8	2.0	0.8	0.4	0.4	1.2	--	--
Other inpatient health facilities	100.0	84.7	6.0	2.1	1.0	1.5	0.5	0.8	0.9	2.5
Mental retardation	100.0	72.5	8.9	3.5	2.1	3.1	0.9	1.5	2.1	5.5
Other	100.0	94.8	3.5	1.0	0.2	0.2	0.2	0.2	--	--

From: *Health Resources Statistics*, The National Center for Health Statistics, U.S. Department of Health, Education, and Welfare, Public Health Service, Health Services and Mental Health Administration, 1968, p. 22.

Table 2.5. Inpatient health facilities, residents, and full-time employees, by type, 1967

Type of facility	Facilities	Residents	Full-time employees
All facilities	30,586	2,445,422	2,561,997
Short-stay hospitals	6,830	676,719	1,583,641
General	6,508	655,603	1,545,270
Specialty	331	21,116	38,371
Long-stay hospitals	1,308	664,210	431,210
General	177	72,803	90,315
Psychiatric	473	499,764	251,885
Geriatric and chronic	307	51,561	45,477
Tuberculosis	166	24,089	24,572
Other	185	15,993	18,961
Nursing care and related homes	19,141	756,239	383,158
Nursing care	10,636	534,721	301,498
Personal care with nursing care	3,853	161,276	63,800
Personal care without nursing care	4,396	56,649	16,361
Domiciliary care	256	3,593	1,499
Other inpatient health facilities	3,298	348,254	163,988
Mental retardation	1,486	218,871	113,098
Other	1,812	129,383	50,890

From: *Health Resources Statistics*, The National Center for Health Statistics, U. S. Department of Health, Education and Welfare, Public Health Service, Health Services and Mental Health Administration, 1968, p. 226.

2.8 The number of beds in 15 hospitals on a specified day is given as: 172, 300, 285, 250, 317, 600, 550, 408, 612, 198, 400, 300, 519, 657, 250.

Are these observations measurements, or classifications with only one class (counts), or a classification with more than one class? Round off each observation to the nearest 50 beds and count the number falling into each class. What term describes the resulting table?

2.9 Two nurses, working in the same ward of the same hospital, wish to compile information showing whether they lose weight more often on the day shift or on the night shift. A "loss of weight" was considered in the study as anything above one pound lost during work hours. The nurses took the following data over a period of 14 working days:

Nurse 1		*Nurse 2*	
Shift	Wt. Loss	Shift	Wt. Loss
Night	Yes	Night	No
Day	No	Night	No
Night	Yes	Night	Yes
Night	Yes	Day	Yes
Day	No	Day	Yes
Day	Yes	Night	No
Night	No	Night	No
Night	Yes	Day	Yes
Day	No	Day	Yes
Night	No	Night	Yes
Day	No	Day	No
Day	No	Night	Yes
Day	No	Night	No
Night	Yes	Day	Yes

a) Summarize the data in a three-way table.
b) Find the relative frequency of nights of weight loss for *both* nurses compared to total number of night shifts worked.
c) Find the same relative frequency for *each* nurse.

2.10 The total body weight of a newborn child is typically distributed as follows: musculature, 25.0%; skin, 19.7%; ligamentous skeleton, 17.0%; brain, cord, and eyeballs, 13.4%; viscera, 11.1%; remainder, 13.8%. Why is this not a statistical frequency table?

2.11 Of those persons 65 years of age and over with activity limitation who reported selected chronic conditions as the cause of their limitation, 21.8% gave heart conditions as the cause, 20.7% gave arthritis and rheumatism, 9.5% gave visual impairments, 8.3% gave hypertension without heart involvement, 5.8% gave mental nervous conditions. Why is this not a statistical frequency table?

LITERATURE CITED

Dixon, W. J., and F. J. Massey. 1957. Introduction to Statistical Analysis. McGraw-Hill Book Company, New York.

Ford, C. E., P. A. Jacobs, and L. G. Lajtha. 1958. Human Somatic Chromosomes. Nature 181:4623, 1965.

Mainland, D. 1964. Elementary Medical Statistics, 2nd Ed. W. B. Saunders Company, Philadelphia.

FURTHER READING

Bennett, A. C. 1964. Methods Improvement in Hospitals. J. B. Lippincott Co., Philadelphia.

Epstein, L. I. 1958. Nomography. Interscience Publishers Inc., New York.

3
Rates, Ratios, and Indices

3.1 INTRODUCTION

Original observations have been described as either measurements or classifications. Although it is advisable, where possible, to work from the basic observations, it often happens that the raw data are already transformed in some way. Thus, taking logarithms of a measure is a transformation of the data. (It is impossible to take logarithms of a blood group or other classification variable.) Frequencies of grouped measurements or of a classification may be presented as relative frequencies or as percentages. The transformation of counts to proportions or percentages so that all the values add up to one (or 100%) is often used to facilitate comparison of frequency distributions. For example, the distribution of length of stay in days for the inpatients of two hospitals can more readily be compared if reduced to percentages. It is also convenient to express a measure of a component of a whole as a percentage of that whole (e.g., weight of the head as a percentage of total body weight; cost of surgical procedures [where appropriate] as a percentage of total bill, number of women in child-bearing years as a percentage of the total number of women in that community).

3.2 RATES

A **rate** is an extension of the concept of a percentage to bases other than 100. Thus, the birth rate may be stated as the number of children born in a given year per 1000 residents in a given area.

Generally this is of the order of 20 per 1000 (which is, of course, just another way of expressing 2%). Two other aspects of rates are apparent from this example. One is that a rate can allow for multiple events per unit item; i.e., a women having two children in a year is counted twice. Similarly, a man having three attacks of influenza in a year is counted three times in calculating the influenza incidence rate, i.e., the number of influenza attacks in a given population in a given period divided by the number of individuals in that population in that period. Thus, to return to our original example, the birth rate is different from the percentage of women who delivered a child in the year (in this, a woman with two births is counted only once).

It is difficult to define the size of the population at risk, because the number of people in a community changes throughout the year. Generally the size of the population at the midpoint of the period is used as the denominator. The population at risk of experiencing the event (birth, influenza) must be defined in time (generally a year in vital statistics) and in space (generally an area for which population size is known or can be estimated). The percentage of beds in a certain hospital occupied at 9 A.M. on a given Monday morning gives a bed occupancy rate that satisfies these requirements concerning the definition of time and place of the population (in this case of beds). Rates used in various fields are defined in the appropriate texts. (See citations under "Further Reading" at the end of this chapter.)

3.3 RATIOS AND INDICES

Most so-called indices are nothing more than ratios; i.e., two associated attributes are measured or counted (generally on the same item) and one is divided by the other to give a decimal number, usually expressed as a percentage. Thus, the obesity index is the ratio of body weight to body volume, and the vital index is simply the ratio of the number of births to the number of deaths in a given community in a given period. Occasionally, one or more of the observations is first transformed; e.g., the ponderal index (the cube root of body weight divided by the person's height) is used instead of body weight, or the pH factor, an index of acidity or alkalinity, is defined as the logarithm of the reciprocal of hydrogen ion concentration in gram molecules per liter of solution. The word **index** is properly applied to statistics that appear to be rates but that, unlike rates, do not describe the number of events occurring in a defined population. Thus, the number of hospital beds per 100,000 of the population or per hospital is an index, not a rate. Similarly the number of personnel per 100 beds is an index not a rate.

Indices that are weighted sums occur when there are a number of responses to be summarized. These are of the form Σwy where w represents the relative weight. Examples occur in diagnostic indices, as in the clinical diagnosis of thyrotoxicosis (Crooks, Murray, and Wayne, 1959), or in the diagnosis of rheumatoid arthritis (Mainland, 1964). Another example is the combination of standard scores of medical students (Kilpatrick, 1971). The tendency to score subjective impressions arbitrarily leads to pseudo-quantification. In the process of adding such scores, much information is lost. Moreover, an additive combination is not necessarily the best, because of the nonindependence of some signs or symptoms. The determination of weights may be also made on an extremely ad hoc basis. Thus, it is often better to use a multiple classification or, if the responses are measured, to use multivariate techniques, which, with the advent of fast digital computers, are becoming increasingly practicable.

Indices of the form $\Sigma w(y/x)$ or $\Sigma wy/\Sigma wx$ also occur. These are weighted sums of ratios or the ratios of two weighted sums. An example of the first occurs in a retrospective study of births in which a mean ratio of placenta weight (PW) to birth weight (BW) was used. This might be expressed as $\Sigma \, (PW/BW)$ divided by $n,$ the number of births. The index formed from the ratio of two weighted sums is best exemplified by the Standardized Mortality ratio (SMR). This compares the mortality in an occupational or other specified group to the mortality in a standard population. The most common misuse of this index is to form the ratio of two SMR's, which has little meaning or justification since the weighting systems in the two SMR's are likely to be different (Kilpatrick, 1963).

There are other indices that are used to estimate some variable incapable of direct measure. Thus, Rohrer's index is an estimate of the nutritional status of the individual and is calculated by dividing weight in grams by the cube of the height in centimeters. The Q-index (Glaser, 1969) is an attempt to measure the importance of a particular disease to the health of a community, and is defined as

$$Q = MDP + \frac{LAK_1}{N} + \frac{BK_1}{N} ,$$

where M = health ratio, D = crude death rate, P = factor for average age at death, L = length of hospital stay, A = number of inpatient days, N = population size, B = number of outpatient days, and K_1, K_2 are constants.

Figure 3.1. Number of work-loss days per currently employed person per year, by occupation group. (From *Disability Days, United States, July 1961–June 1962*, The National Center for Health Statistics, U. S. Public Health Service Publication No. 1000, Ser. 10, No. 4, p. 8.)

Indices are used in all aspects of health care. There are 125 indices listed in *Dorland's Illustrated Medical Dictionary* (1965). The dental profession similarly has coined many indices (see, for example, the Orthodontic Treatment Priority Index [Grainger, 1967] and the Simplified Oral Hygiene Index [Greene and Vermillion, 1964]). The American Hospital Association publishes annual indices by which hospital administrators can judge how deviant their hospital is from the norm in various aspects of health services. Public health workers depend on mortality and morbidity indices to measure the effectiveness of their programs. A good example of the use of rates is given by "The Facts of Life and Death" (Anonymous, 1963) and by the annual reports of the health departments in many regions.

These rates and indices may be tabulated against other variables. Figure 3.1 presents work-loss days per currently employed

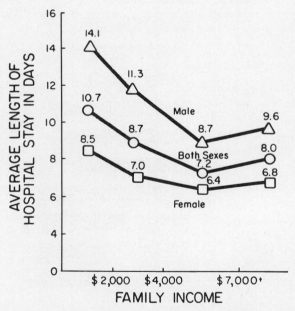

Figure 3.2. Average length of stay in short-stay hospitals, by sex and family income. (From *Medical Care, Health Status, and Family Income, United States,* The National Center for Health Statistics, U. S. Public Health Service Publication No. 1000, Ser. 10, No. 9, p. 14.)

person per year by occupation of the persons concerned. This figure, therefore, shows for each occupation listed the total number of days of work lost divided by the number of persons in that category and by the number of years over which the data were collected. Note that if the data referred to a given year this variable would be simply the average (mean) number of work days lost in each occupational group. This should explain why Figure 3.1 is not a frequency table or histogram.

Figure 3.2 is basically the same as Figure 3.1 in that averages are displayed (for hospitalized individuals by family income and sex).

EXERCISES

3.1 Classify each of the following as a ratio or rate:
number of employees per 100 hospital beds,
number of births per number of deaths,
number of deaths from typhoid per number of cases of typhoid,
number of deaths per number in the population.

3.2 Why is Figure 3.1 not a histogram?

3.3 On how many separate points are the lines in Figure 3.2 based? How many of these can be derived from the others?

LITERATURE CITED

Anonymous. 1963. The Facts of Life and Death. Selected Statistics on the Nation's Health and People. Public Health Service Publication 600. U.S. Government Printing Office, Washington.

Crooks, J., I. P. C. Murray, and E. J. Wayne. 1959. Statistical Methods Applied to the Clinical Diagnosis of Thyrotoxicosis. Quart. J. Med. 28(10):211–234.

Dorland's Illustrated Medical Dictionary. 1965. 24th Ed. W. B. Saunders Company, Philadelphia.

Glaser, J. 1969. More Basic Tools. *In* A Teacher's Guide for Public Health Science. Texas Women's University, Houston.

Grainger, R. M. 1967. Orthodontic Treatment Priority Index. N.C.H.S. Ser. 2, No. 25, U.S. Government Printing Office, Washington.

Greene, J. C., and R. Vermillion, Jr. 1964. The Simplified Oral Hygiene Index. J. Amer. Dent. Ass. 68:7–13.

Kilpatrick, S. J. 1963. Mortality Comparisons in Socio-Economic Groups. Appl. Statist. 12(2):65.

Kilpatrick, S. J. 1971. Alternative Methods of Grading One or More Multiple Choice Examinations. Medical College of Virginia Quarterly 7(1):4—9.

Mainland, D. 1964. Elementary Medical Statistics. 2nd Ed. W. B. Saunders Company, Philadephia.

FURTHER READING

Benjamin, B. 1968. Health and Vital Statistics. Allen & Unwin Ltd., London.

Commission on Hospital Care. 1957. Hospital Care in the United States. Harvard University Press, Cambridge.

Nuffield Provincial Hospitals Trust. 1960. Studies in the Functions and Design of Hospitals. Oxford University Press, London.

Sandler, H. C., and S. S. Stahl. 1959. Measurement of Periodontal Disease Prevalence. J. Amer. Dent. Ass. 58:93—97.

4

Epidemiology and the Design of Surveys

4.1 INTRODUCTION

The meaning of the word **epidemiology** has grown to include much more than the study of epidemics. Now the word is applied to studies of populations (both human and animal) in a given environment. These studies attempt to discover the etiology (causes) of diseases. The method used in these epidemiological studies is to seek associations between some factor in the environment and the disease in question. Since generally the variables are classifications (sick, well; present, absent) these associations are sought in tabulated data, often in the form of multiway tables. The information may be collected for an entire community (a census) as in the Framingham Study of heart disease or the Rhonda Valley Study of blood pressure or, more generally, by selecting (sampling) a small fraction of the population and collecting from the sampled individuals data in which associations are tested. Sampling surveys are called **analytical surveys** when the associations between the variables are the principal interest of the survey. In the health services, the etiology of disease is of less importance as a research interest than is a study of the workings of the system. The methods of epidemiology and sampling surveys are, however, very relevant to statistical research in the health sciences.

Censuses and surveys of health information are made to describe, study, and optimize the system. The description of a health care system is straightforward and is covered in previous chapters by such methods as statistical reduction of data, tabulation, graphing, calculation of rates and indices, etc. To study a health care system, whether it be a nursing home, an outpatient service, or a prepaid medical plan, we need to investigate the relationships among the variables. We may wish to study the relationship in a given hospital between demand for beds and the cost of providing these, or the relationships among tooth decay, mottling, and fluoride concentration in the drinking water, or the relationship between spacing of births and the economic or educational level of the family. It is generally accepted that relationships exist between variables in these sets, but these are complex and not readily reduced to simple formulas. However, if a relationship is known to exist and to follow a certain form, we can predict what will happen if the level of one of the variables is changed and so discover the optimal "settings" for the determinants of the system. The preventive measure of adding fluoride to drinking water is a good example of how communities came independently to accept the relationship between fluoride and dental caries. In considering any problem affecting the health of the population one should also consider its effects upon and its relationships to the remainder of the environment. For example, the opponents of adding fluoride to the drinking water serve the useful purpose of reminding us of the dangers of official control over one of the basic necessities of life and the possibility that this power might be abused. Again, the installation of sewage lines in cities has undoubtedly raised the level of health of urban inhabitants but we must now begin to consider the deleterious effects that dumping raw sewage into rivers may have on the people who live downstream as well as the effects on the river itself and its inhabitants.

The discovery of an association is no guarantee that the relationship is one of simple cause-and-effect. It has never been proved conclusively that cigarette smoking causes lung cancer in man. However, many relationships are readily accepted as cause-and-effect yet causality has never been proved conclusively. Although it is difficult to experiment rigorously in the health care fields, it is possible to try various solutions and see whether they work. If a given solution appears to work in different communities, this can be accepted as empirical proof that the association is cause-and-effect. A distinction should be made between methods arrived at scientifically and any method used by a responsible health professional in providing the best health services. Administrators make decisions without totally understanding the working of their hospitals or the effects of their decisions. Public health doctors also act in the public interest on the basis of incomplete information.

To recapitulate, the object of making a **sample survey** is to investigate the characteristics of a total population without examining every item in the population. Analytical surveys seek to discover relationships between variables in a population in order to reveal the workings of the system under study, whereas descriptive surveys yield estimates or predictions of the characteristics of the population or system studied.

4.2 POPULATION AND SAMPLING UNITS

In a sample survey the population is defined by the investigator as the group to which he wishes to generalize the sample results (or findings). Thus, the sugar concentration in a specimen of blood is of no intrinsic interest, unless this concentration represents the sugar level in all of the patient's blood at that time. The population is therefore defined implicitly as the patient's total blood volume. In many dental indices, the condition of a few surfaces of a few teeth is taken to indicate the condition of the mouth. In this case the population is the teeth in that mouth. In a study showing that on a given date, a sample of hospitals in the United States (of given type and size) had an average of 83% bed occupancy, the implicit population is all institutions in the United States on that date that meet the definition of "hospital." A population then depends on the objective of the investigation and is the total collection of items of interest. It is advisable to explicitly define the population in time and space and with regard to other criteria by which items in the population are recognized.

Confusion often arises between sampling units and measurement units. **Sampling units** are those units comprising the population, since each unit of the population may be selected in a representative sample. One sampling unit, however, may be composed of several **measurement units**, i.e., units that are measured or classified to provide the basic information required. The confusion arises because sampling units and measurement units are synonymous in most situations, e.g., a sample of patients. The difference between sampling units and measurement units can be seen in household surveys where a population of households is sampled but measurements are made on the members of the household to get total family income, say, or to estimate the nutritional status of the family by measuring skin-fold thickness of each individual in the family. In a study of optimal architectural design of hospitals a sample of wards may be taken, but measurements may be made on the amount of walking done by each nurse on duty on each ward.

In order to select the sample, a list or frame of all the sampling units in the population should be available. With such a list, the unambiguous definition of the population is simply those units on the list. Electoral roles, census tracts of households, lists of subscribers to health plans, or directories such as the telephone directory are used to define populations. The availability of such lists saves a great deal of time and labor provided the investigator is prepared to amend the definition of his population to those units on the available list. It is not always possible to construct a frame or list. For example, the population of interest might be conceptual or ill-defined (mankind, including past and future members of the human species; patients with a given condition; people using a certain medical facility; all carcinogenic substances, etc.). Although the real population of interest may be so large that it is difficult to define it precisely, it is generally better to restrict the survey to give a valid generalization of a limited or restricted population or subpopulation. This allows the reader the option to generalize to the wider population at his own risk. Thus, if a study has shown that a certain dose of aspirin was beneficial in treating a sample of 13 female patients with rheumatoid arthritis, the physician who uses this study as a basis for treating male patients with rheumatoid arthritis with aspirin does so because of his own generalization, not because of those of the investigator. Limited resources also dictate that the population of interest be reduced to manageable size. Thus, a survey by a student collecting information for a thesis on hospitals may have to be restricted to a particular state, if the survey calls for a personal visit to each hospital in the sample. Of course, the alternative, a nationwide survey of hospitals by mail, should also be considered. A compromise between the quality of the sample data and the size of the population has to be reached.

4.3 USE OF AUXILIARY INFORMATION IN SAMPLING

Often a list or frame of the sampling units in a population is available with, or can be made to include, auxiliary information, i.e., additional information beyond that needed to identify the units. This information may be used in two ways—in **stratifying** the population and in checking the representativeness of the sample. Consider a telephone directory and assume that we delete all business listings. The remaining information is simply a list of the names and addresses of subscribers (excluding those with unlisted numbers) and may be considered in terms of the above definition to contain no auxiliary information. However, we may group subscribers by area of residence (either by their addresses or their telephone prefixes). Also, we can classify names listed as belonging to males, females, or sex unknown, and we can further classify to some extent by titles used in the listing (M.D., Rev., Esq., etc.) and by households (same surname, same address). Nothing is gained, however, by subdividing the subscribers into subpopulations on the basis of this information unless one of the variables of interest in the survey is related to these subdivisions. For example, we may know beforehand that in an attitudinal study of Medicare, doctors' attitudes are different from those of the rest of the public, that men differ from women in their attitudes to cigarette smoking, or that residents in the core city differ from residents in the suburbs with regard to attitudes toward contraception. If this knowledge is available and relevant to our study, i.e., that occupation is related to health care attitudes, that sex is related to the respondent's opinion on cigarette smoking, etc., we should divide the entries in the telephone directory into groups according to these classifications. By sampling separately from each of these subgroups, we can insure that the sample is representative of the total population of listed subscribers. If the sample is not representative, we can adjust our estimates to allow for, say, an excess of M.D.'s in the sample compared with the population. We can also combine the separate estimates from the various subgroups in any desired proportion, thus giving an estimate for all adult residents in the area (which is not the same as the population of listed telephone subscribers) or giving an estimate for a greater area than that represented by the directory, say, the state. This assumes, however, that with regard to the examples above, subscribers in this area are typical of subscribers in the remainder of the area or state in their attitudes towards Medicare, cigarette smoking, and contraceptives.

A second use to which ancillary information on the sampling units of a population may be put is to check whether the selected sample is representative of the population. If, say, the ages of a given group of patients are known and 10% of these are taken as a sample, it is helpful to know the ages of the 10% sampled and to check whether there is approximately the same proportion of old people in the sample as in the population, etc. This, of course, does not guarantee that the sample information is identical with or even similar to that for the whole group or population except with regard to age. An old movie once suggested the existence of a typical town in which the characteristics of the inhabitants were, on an average, exactly those of the population of the United States at the time—same proportion of old and young, male and female, black and white, etc. Even if this community did exist there would be no guarantee that the inhabitants' attitudes on politics, religion, sex, health care, or any other topic would be typical of the United States. In other words, because a sample is like the population from which it is drawn in one respect, there is no reason to believe that it is similar to the population in any other respect.

4.4 SURVEY INSTRUMENTS AND PILOT STUDIES

Although they are outside the scope of this text, a few generalizations about survey instruments may be useful. The term **survey**

instrument occurs most frequently in the behavioral sciences, where the survey is an attempt to elicit information from a given population in reference to some concept that is imprecisely defined but assumed to exist. Thus, the concept of intelligence is difficult to define precisely but is still generally accepted. In a survey of intelligence, a specific I.Q. test may be administered and the scores used as an indirect measure of intelligence. In this case, the I.Q. test serves as the survey instrument used to measure intelligence. In a public health survey of nutrition, multiple measures may be made (on diet, skin-fold thickness, etc.) and combined into an index of nutrition to serve as a survey instrument. In a study of unwanted pregnancy, a knowledge, attitude, and practice (KAP) survey may be made on contraceptives. The survey will elicit from the respondents what they know about contraceptives, what their attitudes are, and to what extent they practice contraception. Thus, it is clear that a concept that is difficult to measure (or classify) is replaced by a battery of simpler questions that can be answered. The danger in the use of an indirect survey instrument is that we equate the survey instrument with the concept being estimated. Those who maintain that there is no evidence that one race is more intelligent than another do so largely on the ground that intelligence is immeasurable and that the I.Q. tests used are biased in favor of the culture of the majority race. The development of sensitive and accurate survey instruments is a valid area of research in all disciplines of the health care field where concepts are diffuse but meaningful, as, for example, in the health of the community.

Pilot studies may be used to test proposed survey instruments. A pilot study is a small-scale preliminary study designed to validate certain crucial assumptions about the proposed investigation. Thus, in the context of surveys, a pilot study is a very small sample survey performed before the main survey in order to evaluate the mechanisms of the survey (is it feasible to interview all members of a sample? is the questionnaire understood by the respondents?), to estimate the response rate of the survey (if the pilot indicates that only 50% of those receiving a mailed questionnaire will return it within 30 days perhaps some other method of contacting potential respondents should be used since a survey with only a 50% response is of little value), and to test the survey instrument to be used (by checking pilot results against known facts). In other words, in a pilot study, all aspects of the investigation (here, a survey) are carried out on a small scale in order to reveal methodological difficulties in the generation, analysis, and interpretation of information.

4.5 TYPES OF SAMPLING

The most natural and easiest methods of selecting a sample are generally not the best. A "convenient" sample is one selected in the easiest way for that situation, e.g., interview the first ten nurses that one meets in the corridors of a hospital. A "batch" sample is one in which the members of the sample fall together in space and time; e.g., the hospital bills of patients discharged on a given day is a batch sample of the total population of discharged patients' bills. A "batch" sample is thus often also a "convenient" sample. Other frequent methods of selecting members of a population into a sample are systematic sampling, pseudo-random sampling, and inverse sampling.

Systematic sampling consists of selecting every kth item in the population, e.g., enumerating or listing all beds in a hospital and selecting every fifth bed to give a 20% sample. Pseudo-random sampling occurs when the investigator claims to have selected a sample at random, but has, in fact, selected items from the population, the selection being determined by a number of unknown forces; e.g., "a random sample of patients with colitis was treated by a new method" may mean that the physician directing the clinical trial on colitis used available patients whom, he felt, it was ethical to treat in a new manner. Moreover, he believes that these patients are representative of all patients with colitis. The statement that three mice were chosen at random from a cage of ten may simply mean that the medical scientist put his hand into a cage three times, each time removing the first animal he encountered.

Inverse sampling occurs when items are selected until a predetermined number have been collected, each of which has the attribute in question. This approach is useful when studying conditions that occur rarely. For example, in studying the relative importance of accidents in the home as a cause of death among men aged from 25 to 45 years, death certificates may be examined until a certain number of these reveal that death was caused by fatal accidents at home. This insures that the sample includes a given number of deaths from this cause.

Probability sampling refers to sampling schemes in which the probability of selection of each item in the population can be specified. The most widely known and the simplest type of probability sampling is random sampling, often known as "simple random sampling." In simple random sampling the items in the population are numbered 1, 2, . . . , etc. Then the requisite number of values are taken from a table of random numbers such as Table 4.1 and items with these numbers are selected into the sample. By the use of random number tables, each item in the population has the same chance of being selected as any other item. If the sample is small compared to the population, we may assume that sampling with or without replacement gives effectively the same results. The composition of a simple random sample is determined strictly by chance. Infrequently the sample may be unrepresentative, i.e., if we selected health insurance claims in a strictly random way, we might inadvertently select all claims for medical treatment provided by one doctor or all claims of the same type, say, surgical procedures. If the population is divided into subpopulations or subgroups, it seems reasonable to require the same **sampling fraction** of each group. Thus, if we wanted a 10% sample of health insurance claims made by residents in a given city, it might be reasonable to stratify the population of claims according to the provider of health care (hospitals, group practices, individual physicians, etc.), and to insist that 10% of the claims originating from each health care unit be taken into the sample. While apparently reasonable, stratified sampling is called for only if the variable of interest, say, the amount of the bill, varies according to which group provided the service. In the current example there is an association between the amount of the bill and the organizational unit of health care, since, in general, bills from hospital-based physicians tend to be higher than bills from office-based physicians. This is a reflection only on the

Table 4.1. Random sample numbers

```
1 5 9 6    3 0 6 9    7 9 0 6    6 6 5 6    5 2 9 8
4 9 5 1    6 9 9 3    5 2 4 3    6 3 7 5    5 0 8 8
9 8 6 7    0 3 9 9    6 7 4 1    1 5 7 9    7 5 5 2
2 6 7 0    7 9 6 9    2 9 0 9    8 7 0 5    0 1 8 8
5 8 0 8    4 3 2 9    6 6 8 1    9 8 5 2    9 4 5 8

8 2 9 8    1 1 2 5    9 1 5 3    9 5 1 7    1 4 8 1
3 1 1 7    0 2 3 9    0 7 7 0    8 0 3 4    9 9 7 8
2 3 5 8    1 9 7 9    1 1 2 0    3 1 0 9    1 1 6 9
0 0 3 9    4 4 6 1    8 6 7 4    5 2 9 6    8 1 1 1
2 4 0 0    4 9 7 1    0 4 6 4    1 8 4 9    7 0 5 5

5 9 8 9    6 7 4 9    8 8 3 2    2 7 6 0    5 2 2 0
0 9 9 6    0 8 5 1    9 6 5 9    7 1 0 7    0 1 2 1
6 9 0 9    4 9 7 1    4 0 8 7    4 7 8 3    9 6 9 4
7 8 4 1    5 9 3 0    8 1 5 7    0 1 3 0    8 8 1 8
4 8 9 1    6 2 2 3    9 2 5 2    9 2 5 9    2 1 7 4

1 0 3 6    9 1 3 3    5 4 0 7    1 7 3 4    5 1 1 4
9 1 4 0    7 8 9 6    0 8 8 1    7 0 6 4    5 8 6 2
1 2 8 1    8 6 1 3    3 4 3 1    0 1 0 4    0 6 8 9
9 4 2 6    3 8 1 9    5 7 6 1    8 0 1 9    3 6 3 7
9 1 5 6    4 8 6 7    9 2 6 9    6 1 4 9    4 4 7 1

7 6 1 1    3 5 0 8    9 1 8 2    1 7 3 8    5 7 7 2
5 0 4 5    3 5 2 4    8 2 5 0    4 0 5 3    4 3 4 3
5 3 0 2    2 6 6 0    1 6 1 8    1 5 9 5    0 3 4 4
3 6 8 9    5 0 2 8    6 3 0 2    4 5 5 2    9 5 1 3
0 1 4 8    2 4 4 9    5 4 9 1    2 6 0 7    5 4 2 5

2 8 8 1    7 8 3 5    1 1 8 8    1 7 0 5    2 2 5 4
7 9 2 4    5 5 0 5    0 4 3 2    3 1 0 1    0 9 9 5
1 9 8 0    8 4 2 0    7 2 2 5    8 2 9 2    2 5 5 7
0 9 8 7    2 4 6 7    1 8 2 0    3 6 9 4    7 6 5 0
7 5 5 8    5 5 6 3    2 4 3 1    0 1 4 4    0 0 9 9

9 1 4 9    1 0 8 1    0 4 2 6    4 2 0 1    1 9 8 4
6 8 3 0    6 8 6 6    0 0 3 2    9 7 7 7    1 5 9 9
3 6 9 0    4 6 3 4    8 8 5 0    7 2 5 7    1 5 2 3
6 3 1 1    0 0 7 3    2 7 0 6    0 5 5 8    1 8 3 1
4 5 0 0    1 6 3 5    9 6 5 2    3 8 5 0    3 0 0 5
```

acuteness and gravity of the patient's condition rather than on the practice of medicine. Conversely, we could stratify a year's claims according to the month of billing. It is debatable whether there is any significant variation in average health care bills from month to month, so it is doubtful that a sample stratified by month would give a better estimate of the average amount of a medical bill that year than a simple random sample. Finally, we can alter the sampling fraction in different strata so that small but relevant strata are well represented. Thus, if we had four hospitals and 400 family practitioners we could have the following:

Large hospital	—	10% sample of patients' bills
Small hospital	—	20% sample of patients' bills
Two specialized hospitals	—	50% sample of patients' bills
100 family practitioners randomly selected out of a total of 400.	—	5% sample of patients' bills

If the sampling fraction is known for each stratum, an overall estimate can be formed by combining the separate estimates from each stratum in accordance with the number of items in the population that the sample represents.

Note that the order in which these sampling methods have been presented corresponds roughly to a required increase in background information on the population. In convenience, batch, or pseudo-random sampling, the investigator does not have to enumerate or list the items in the population, whereas in the latter methods, simple random and stratified random sampling, a frame, or list, of the population must be available. In the case of stratified sampling we also need to be able to classify the population items with reference to one or more ancillary variables. The art of making sample surveys is knowing how to exploit all the information one has about the population or in getting easily accessible auxiliary information that is relevant to the variables of interest.

4.6 SIZE OF SAMPLES

The question most frequently asked of statisticians is "What size should my sample be?" To answer it the person designing the survey has to know which population is to be sampled, as well as the number and characteristics of the variables of interest. He must know for each measure, the mean and standard deviation, and the percentage falling into each class for each classification. Thus, it appears that the optimal sample size can be specified only after the survey has been done. This is where pilot surveys are helpful in providing estimates for the average level of each response and some idea of the variation from one item to another. The larger the sample the more accurate the estimate of the population will be, and the more sensitive the survey in detecting associations among factors or variables. Paradoxically, nearly the same accuracy is achieved in samples of the same size even though these samples may be drawn from populations of vastly different sizes. Thus a sample of 50 beds from a 350-bed hospital may have the same accuracy as a sample of 50 hospitals from the approximately 7,000 hospitals in the United States.

4.7 PROBLEM OF NONRESPONSE

Having determined the items to be examined to provide the sample data, one often finds it impossible to obtain a value for certain items. This is because some individuals may refuse to answer a questionnaire, some houses may be empty, some animals may die, some observations may be lost, etc. Every effort should be made to minimize the proportion of nonresponses, since the findings of a survey with a high proportion of nonresponders may be invalid. To calculate the effect of nonresponses on a survey estimate, it is wise to calculate what the estimate would be if all nonresponders responded first one way and then the other way. For example, assume that in a hypothetical survey of discharged patients' attitudes toward the quality of care provided during their last hospitalization, a population of 1,512 patients discharged in the previous year was identified and attempts were made to elicit the attitudes of 150 randomly selected ex-patients. Let us assume that questionnaires were mailed to their last known addresses and replies were received (after repeated mailings) from 121. This is a response rate of 81%. Let us say that of these 121 replies 97 reported favorable and 24 unfavorable attitudes toward the quality of care. If we assume that the reason for nonresponse was not related to the ex-patients' attitudes, then we can say that 24 out of 121 or 20% were dissatisfied with the standard of care provided and apply this to the whole population of 1,512 discharged patients. However, it is unreasonable to assume that lack of response is unconnected with the discharged patients' attitudes. One could argue that satisfied ex-patients would be more likely not to respond than irate ex-patients or that nonresponse was due to the death of the discharged patient, which in turn may be due to an inferior standard of care. The point is that we do not know what caused the nonresponse so we assume the worst (all nonresponders dissatisfied) and the best (all nonresponders satisfied). We now are able to bracket our figure of 20% dissatisfied with a possible maximum of

$$\frac{24 + 29}{150} = \frac{53}{150} = 35\%$$

and a possible minimum of

$$\frac{24 + 0}{150} = \frac{24}{150} = 16\%.$$

Thus, because of nonresponse the nonsampling range of error in our estimate is from 16% to 35%. Unfortunately this approach is inappropriate if the variable is a classification with more than two categories or is a measure with a large range of possible results.

4.8 PROBLEM OF INCOMPLETE INFORMATION

Surveys generate information on many variables. Generally many responses are required from the sampled individual or item. This leads to the situation where an overall response is available from an individual but some questions are unanswered. In terms of single variables we may use the approach in the above section of nonresponse, calculating high and low estimates when the variable is a classification with two groups. Otherwise we are forced to use the available information on the assumption (often tenuous) that the reason for the missing value is unconnected to its value. A further complication is that the effective sample size (i.e., the number of values for each variable) will differ from one variable to another. Missing observations are more of a problem when the survey is analytical, i.e., when the relationship between the variables is of interest. Thus, if in the hypothetical survey of ex-patients' attitudes toward hospital care, we were interested in studying the relationship between one's religious denomination and his attitude, and the respondents' religious affiliation has not been reported, we would have to omit that association from the investigation. Although one might turn to other sources of information when some of the questions are unanswered, this is often either impractical or unethical.

4.9 ERRORS AND INCONSISTENCIES IN THE DATA

In surveys the investigator is heavily dependent on others for the generation of the data. This means that errors in communication can arise, with the result that some responses may be useless and must be omitted from subsequent analysis. Deliberate errors may arise in a response to a question when the respondent is trying to hide something from the investigator. Errors can also arise in transcribing, coding, and key punching the information. For example, a zero may be punched when an observation is missing. An error arises if another response has a true zero reading and the two meanings of zero get confused in analysis. Thus in a survey of the amount of federal financial support of professional training, volunteer workers included in the sample may answer "−" or N.A. (not applicable). If both are coded 0 (zero), the proportion of health care workers who had no federal assistance in their training will be inflated. In a small survey where the investigator has an intimate knowledge of the data, inconsistencies can be spotted visually. In large computer-based surveys, it is advisable to program the computer to check for inconsistencies. These checks follow common-sense rules based on a knowledge of the type of information gathered. Thus those returns of the 1961 Census in England that showed that a mother had borne more than 19 children (Benjamin, 1960) were returned by the computer for checking. Other incongruities may be defined and appropriate action taken. These include imputation, i.e., substituting an imputed observation for one clearly wrong, such as a future year of marriage or other event.

4.10 ANALYSIS OF SURVEY DATA

Sample data may be condensed to means, proportions, and cross-tabulations of one variable against another. Variation in sample measures may be explained by the range of sample values or the standard deviation. These sample statistics are used to estimate the values of the corresponding population statistics. Thus, if a random sample of ten members of a graduating class of hospital administrators was polled two years after graduation and the mean income was calculated for the ten respondents, this value could be used as the estimated population mean of the whole class of graduating students. Likewise, if these ten were asked to name their area of specialization and two replied "accounting," we could use this sample proportion to estimate the proportion of graduates in the population who were specializing in "accounting." This type of survey is purely descriptive. However, we may be interested in predicting the average income of future graduates of schools of hospital administration and in predicting the number or proportion of these graduates specializing in "accounting." This could be done if a series of such surveys were carried out in successive years. Thus the change in estimated average income from one year to the next might suggest a trend that, if continued, would give a prediction for future graduates. Similarly, if in three successive annual surveys 0/10, 1/10, 2/10 of the population indicated "accounting" as a speciality, it would be reasonable to assume that this increase in the proportion specializing in accounting might continue. Regression analysis and time series analysis (Chapter 11) are used to predict future averages and proportions.

Estimates from one survey may be compared with those of other surveys of similar nature made by different investigators at different times and in different places. Again, in stratified surveys, the investigator may wish to compare the response in one stratum with that in another. In all such comparisons it is not clear whether the differences that are revealed are real or due to change (i.e., **sampling variation**). We need to use statistical tests of significance in order to discriminate, with a given amount of confidence, between real differences and differences due to chance mechanisms arising in the sampling of the population.

Finally, in analytical surveys we are mainly interested in the detection of an association between one variable and another. In this case, too, an apparent association or relationship in sampled data may be due to sampling variation, i.e., a sample survey of 20 babies showed that birth weight decreased as parity increased. The question is, if a larger number of birth weights were tabulated against parity, would the same relationship hold? This question and others like it may be answered by statistical tests of association such as **correlation** and χ^2.

EXERCISES

4.1 What are the difficulties in obtaining a representative sample of the following?
   a) all mothers who will deliver a live child in a given hospital next year,
   b) patients suffering from arthritis, in order to administer a controlled clinical trial of a new treatment,
   c) families registered in a comprehensive health care plan.

4.2 When is it appropriate to take a sample, and when is it necessary to carry out a census?

4.3 Ten hospitals are selected from a list of all registered hospitals in the state and all heads of departments in these hospitals are interviewed regarding the morale of their staffs.
   a) Name the sampling units in this survey,
   b) Name the measurement units in this survey,
   c) Name the population of interest,
   d) Hypothesize what the conclusion of the survey might be.

4.4 An EKG of a given patient is taken. What is the implied population? Why is a random sample of this implied population difficult to get?

4.5 Normal values for systolic blood pressure used by a given physician are based on his study of 30 normal medical students. What implied assumptions is the physician making in using these values?

4.6 What are the advantages and disadvantages of the following?
   a) a pilot study,
   b) a random sample,
   c) an analytical survey to discover whether a high fat diet causes heart failure,
   d) a 10% random sample of all morticians, with a 46% response rate, regarding the pros and cons of cremation.

LITERATURE CITED

Benjamin, B. 1960. Statistical Problems of the 1961 Population Census. J. Roy. Statist. Soc., Ser. A., 123(4):413.

FURTHER READING

Cochran, W. G. 1965. The Planning of Observational Studies of Human Population. J. Roy. Statist. Soc., Ser. A., 128:234.

Hollis, G. G. 1971. Design and Methodology of the 1967 Master Facility Inventory Survey. N.C.H.S. Public Health Service Publication No. 1000:1–9. U.S. Government Printing Office, Washington.

Morris, J. N. 1964. Uses of Epidemiology. 2nd Ed. The Williams & Wilkins Co., Baltimore.

Paul, J. R. 1966. Clinical Epidemiology. Rev. Ed. The University of Chicago Press, Chicago.

Roueche, B. 1953. Eleven Blue Men and Other Narratives of Medical Detection. Berkley Publishing Corporation, New York.

Stuart, A. 1964. Basic Ideas of Scientific Sampling. Hafner Publishing Company Inc., New York.

Taylor, I., and J. Knowelden, Jr. 1964. Principles of Epidemiology. 2nd Ed. Blackwell Scientific Publications Ltd., Oxford.

5

Distributions
Location and Dispersion, Normal Variation

5.1 DISTRIBUTIONS

As we noted above, an excellent method of condensing information is to count the number of times a given value appears. When each value occurs once only, we can still condense the data by using nonoverlapping but contiguous intervals and by counting the number of times values of a variable fall into these intervals. This gives a frequency distribution, from which we can prepare a table or graph of the number of times a certain value occurs. These frequencies may be expressed as relative frequencies, i.e., as percentages of times the variable has values falling into a given class interval.

The times of the day at which children under 14 years of age are involved in pedestrian accidents are given in Table 5.1. Since the hours between 10:00 P.M. and 6:00 A.M. are omitted, it is reasonable to assume that an insignificant percentage of pedestrian accidents occurred during these hours. A graph of this relative frequency distribution is shown in Figure 5.1. Conceptually, a frequency distribution of a continuous variable or measure is thought of as a smooth curve. Such a curve could be achieved by using smaller and smaller class intervals, as in Figure 5.1. Since all child pedestrian accidents are assumed to have occured between

Table 5.1. Frequency of child pedestrian accidents by time of day, Baltimore, Maryland, 1956–1958

Time Interval	Percentage
6:00 - 7:59 A.M.	2.0
8:00 - 9:59	4.0
10:00 - 11:59	12.0
12:00 - 1:59 P.M.	13.5
2:00 - 3:59	24.0
4:00 - 5:59	30.0
6:00 - 7:59	10.5
8:00 - 9:59	4.0
Total	100.0

Figure 5.1. Frequency of child pedestrian accidents by time of day, Baltimore, Maryland, 1956–1958.

6:00 A.M. and 10:00 P.M., the area under the frequency distribution is equal to 100%.

One may think of a frequency distribution of a variable as a description of all the values the variable can have. The distribution will peak at those values that occur frequently and will be low at those values that occur rarely. A frequency distribution, therefore, is a complete description of a continuous variable. It is analogous to a classification associated with a discrete variable. The importance of a frequency distribution is that it describes the variability of the measure as well as its typical values. Variability pervades the health sciences and the information generated by the health services. Too often this variability is overlooked or not taken into consideration. In the provision of health care, attention must be given to the atypical as well as to the typical.

5.2 MEASURES OF LOCATION

Before defining measures of variation, we review and extend our concepts of measures of location, sometimes called measures of central tendency. The most common average used is the mean (so common, in fact, that this is what the layman understands by the word average). The **mean** is the sum of the observations (made on a continuous variable) divided by the number of observations. Arithmetically the mean of $53, $55, $50, $68 and $54 is

$$\$(53 + 55 + 50 + 68 + 54)/5 = \$(280)/5 = \$56.$$

Four of the observations start with 5 so one could save work by splitting each number into 50 and a remainder. Thus, the mean would be calculated as:

$$\$(50 + 3 + 50 + 5 + 50 + 0 + 50 + 18 + 50 + 4)/5 \begin{aligned} &= \$(250 + 30)/5 \\ &= \$250/5 + \$30/5 \\ &= \$50 + \$6 \\ &= \$56. \end{aligned}$$

(Note that, although there are ten numbers in the numerator, we divide by 5 because there are still only five observations.) In this calculation we change the origin from 0 to 50 and convert the original values into amounts in excess of $50 ($3, $5, $0, $18, and $4). The mean of these amounts over $50 is

$$\$(3 + 5 + 0 + 18 + 4)/5 = \$30/5 = \$6,$$

which indicates that the mean is $6 greater than $50, or $56. Note that the value which the mean takes is not necessarily one of the observations. This can result in a mean which is misleading! Consider a maternity ward in which the mean age of the mothers and children is 9.2 years. This is clearly too young to represent maternal ages and too old to represent ages of newborn. In fact, an average should be calculated only when the observations pertain to a homogeneous group. Averages serve no purpose in the description of mixed populations such as mothers and children.

The **median** is the middle value when the observations are arranged in order. The middle value of $50, $53, $54, $55, and $68 is $54. If the number of observations is even, then the median is the mean of the two central observations arranged in order of size. The median, being a middle value, is not influenced by the size of the extreme values. Thus, in the example above, the median of the five observations is unchanged when the value of the largest observation is increased from $68 to $168 or changed to any other value greater than the median, $54. The median is useful, therefore, in describing the center of a distribution that may contain extreme values, for example, hospital income or daily hospital costs.

The **mode** is the value (or values) that occurs most often in a distribution. In the above example, each dollar value occurs once only. Therefore, one might say that each one is a mode or that there is no mode at all, because no value or set of values occurs more often than any other. In Table 5.1 the mode is the time interval 4:00–5:59 P.M., since this interval contains the highest percentage of all pedestrian accidents to children. In the absence of other information, it may be assumed that the mode would occur at 5:00 P.M. (half-way through the most frequently occurring interval, 4:00–5:59 P.M.). The mode is useful when we want to know the most frequently occurring value. For example, at what age do most people first experiment with drugs? What is the most frequent dosage of a given medication? After what period of service do most hospital employees start looking for another job? In all these examples the value that supplies this kind of information is the mode rather than the mean or median.

5.3 NOTATION

It is necessary at this stage to introduce symbols and abbreviations to facilitate the use of the concepts of location and dispersion. For the beginner, notation is often a stumbling block, but it is necessary to permit a clearer description of the subject, to familiarize him with standard practices, and to train him in the use of different kinds of notations. To the executive, it is more important to understand the concept implied by a symbol than it is to know how to derive or calculate a value. In their training, health professionals spend a large portion of time learning the language of their discipline. If they are to make decisions and to lead a team, they must also learn to read reports from financial analysts, manpower experts, operations research workers, statisticians, and data processing experts.

In the formulation of a notation for averages we need six symbols: population mean, median, and mode, and sample mean, median, and mode. We follow the usual practice (Halperin, Hartley, and Hoel, 1965) in using μ for the population mean and $\bar{x}$ for the mean of a sample of x-values. We use μ_{50} and $\bar{x}_{50}$ for the population and sample median, respectively. This is similar to the pharmacological use of an LD_{50}, which signifies a dose that can kill 50% of the animals treated. For the mode we use the symbols μ_o and $\bar{x}_o$. The o is derived from the o in "mode," and is a letter that does not occur in the words "mean" or "median." The student should familiarize himself with these terms so that their use will not confuse him. (See Appendix.)

5.4 MEASURES OF DISPERSION

We are already familiar with the concept of range in measuring the variation in a sample of observations. Since r is generally reserved for the sample correlation coefficient, let us use w for the sample range or width. Then

$$w = \text{maximum value} - \text{minimum value},$$

and in the case of the five observations given above,

$$w = \$68 - \$50 = \$18.$$

It is possible to conceive of the range in a population of values but, since these are often so wide as to be of little interest, no symbol is given for population range.

The second measure of variation is the **standard deviation.** Although it is more common than the range, it is more difficult to define. The sample standard deviation s is calculated as

$$s = \sqrt{\frac{\Sigma(x - \overline{x})^2}{n - 1}}$$

in a sample of n observations on a variable x for which the sample mean is $\overline{x}$. The standard deviation is sometimes called the "root mean square" of deviations from the mean. If we knew the complete population we could calculate the standard deviation as

$$\sigma = \sqrt{\frac{\Sigma(x - \mu)^2}{N}}$$

where N is the size of the population. Note that in order to get an unbiased estimate of σ^2, the population **variance**, we use $(n - 1)$ as a denominator for the sample variance:

$$s^2 = \frac{\Sigma(x - \overline{x})^2}{n - 1}$$

We can use a numerical example to explain how to calculate s. Consider the five observations $53, \$55, \$50, \$68, \$54$. If we call the variable x, the steps in calculating the sample standard deviation are as follows:

Step 1.   Calculate $\overline{x} = \Sigma x / n = \$56.$
Step 2.   Form deviations of the values of x from $\overline{x}$; that is,

$$(53 - 56) = -3, (55 - 56) = -1, (50 - 56) = -6,$$
$$(68 - 56) = 12, (54 - 56) = -2.$$

Note: The sum of these deviations is zero.

Step 3.   Add the squares of the deviations in Step 2:

$(-3)^2 + (-1)^2 + (-6)^2 + (12)^2 + (-2)^2 = 9 + 1 + 36 + 144 + 4 = 194.$

Step 4.   Divide the "sum of squares" in step 3 by $n - 1$ (the sample size minus 1):

$$\frac{194}{5-1} = \frac{194}{4} = 48.50.$$

Step 5.   Take the square root of the result of step 4:

$$s = \sqrt{48.50} = \$6.96.$$

An equivalent formula that is better suited to desk calculators or computers is

$$s = \sqrt{\frac{\Sigma x^2 - (\Sigma x)^2/n}{n-1}}$$

At this stage the concept of a standard deviation is still unformed in the student's mind. His typical questions are: "How did such a complicated concept arise and what does it mean?" The concept of the standard deviation is used in the formulation of the normal distribution and thus it is most meaningful for observations that follow this type of frequency distribution. Likewise, its interpretation can best be described in terms of the normal distribution. Therefore, answers to these (reasonable) questions will be found below in Section 5.5. Note that both the standard deviation and w, the sample range, are in the same units as the basic variable x.

5.5 THE NORMAL DISTRIBUTION

The normal or Gaussian distribution is a theoretical frequency distribution. Its central position in statistics occurs largely because many naturally occurring frequency distributions follow the normal distribution, if only approximately (see Figure 5.2). If it is known that the observations follow a normal distribution, all these observations can be summarized in only two statistics: the population mean and the standard deviation. Thus, if we assert that the

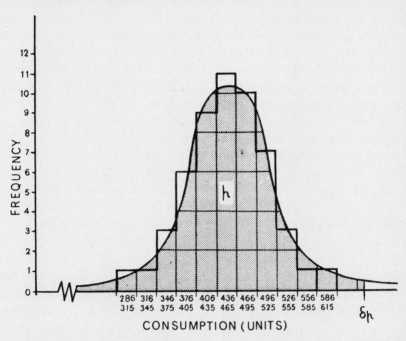

Figure 5.2. Histogram of consumption with normal frequency distribution superimposed. (From *Problems and Progress in Medical Care,* Second Series, G. McLachlan (ed.), p. 190, Fig. 2. Published for the Nuffield Provincial Hospitals Trust by Oxford University Press, 1966.)

heights of white, 18 year-old males in the United States in 1977 follow a normal distribution, we can represent this large population of heights simply by giving the mean height as, say, 68.7 in. and the standard deviation as 2.77 in. This ability to reduce the information contained in a large or infinite number of observations to three facts—the statement that the observations follow a normal distribution and the value of two parameters, the mean and the standard deviation in that distribution—is the ultimate in the condensation of data. The description of the values a continuous variable may take, in terms of the underlying distribution, has motivated much of the past development of statistical theory.

The normal frequency distribution follows a single-peaked, symmetrical curve reducing to zero frequencies at plus and minus infinity, and satisfying other conditions implicit in its formulation.

Not all unimodal symmetrical distributions with an infinite range are normal distributions. However, the methods that are based on the concept of the normal distribution also apply fairly accurately to observations with a nonnormal distribution. In fact, this **robustness** to departures from the normal distribution is another reason why statistical methods, often based on an unvalidated assumption of an underlying normal distribution, are universally applied. Indeed, the paradox arises when a scrupulous investigator with a large amount of data tests these data to see whether they follow a normal distribution. Since often they will not (exactly), the scrupulous investigator will avoid using these techniques based on the normal distribution. In most cases he would be well advised to apply these analytical techniques anyway, since the methods will give nearly the same result if the distribution follows a normal distribution precisely. In a small sample, the situation arises less often, since there is less chance of showing that the distribution of a small sample of observations is not normal. Therefore, statistical methods are usually applied to small samples of data without testing those data for normality.

There is one case, however, that arises quite frequently in small samples of observations, in which a test for normality is useful. This is a test for outliers. An **outlier** is an observation that is so far from the mean of the sample (in standard deviation units) that it is very likely that the value quoted is inaccurate. The evaluation of a possible outlier must be made in terms of a knowledge of the system. If a patient's age were given as 120 years, we would question it. Similarly we would question the statements that a person weighs 450 lb, that a given mother had 32 children, or that a patient had a temperature of 58.4°F. A simple statistical test for outliers in small samples is given in Section 9.6.1.

To evaluate observations in large samples we may apply the following test for outliers. Any observation that is more than three standard deviations from the mean may be an outlier, since there is only one chance in 100 that any observation in a normal distribution will fall outside of plus or minus three standard deviation units from the mean. This assumes, of course, that we know or have estimated the mean and the standard deviation fairly accurately and that the other observations are normally distributed. The use of the formula $\mu \pm 3\sigma$ to provide effective limits for the normal distribution is derived from the property that

$$P(\mu - 3\sigma < x < \mu + 3\sigma) \approx 0.99,$$

where x is any observation chosen at random, and μ and σ are the mean and standard deviation of the normal distribution, and P is probability. Note that, for the normal distribution,

$$P(\mu - 2\sigma < x < \mu + 2\sigma) \approx 0.95,$$

so that approximately 95% and 99% of the normal distribution lie within two and three standard deviations of the mean.

In a small sample of data the presence of an outlier will always increase the standard deviation s calculated for that sample. Thus, we would be misled into thinking that there is more variation in that particular variable or system than there is. Outliers, then, are considered to be freak observations caused by large errors, such as transcribing a number or using an incorrect measurement technique. However, outliers found in a study should be reported so that the reader may decide how to interpret them and how to avoid giving a false image of efficiency in data collection.

EXERCISES

5.1 The mean of a sample of measurements can be calculated by dividing their sum by the number of observations. When the sample size is large, observations having the same value can be combined and the frequency with which each value occurs can be given. In this case the mean is calculated as the sum of the values times their frequency divided by the total frequency. Demonstrate that these two approaches are equivalent by

a) showing that

$$\bar{x} = \frac{\Sigma x}{x} = \sum_{i=1}^{m} f_i x_i \bigg/ \sum_{i=1}^{m} f_i$$

where m = the number of different values of x that occur in the sample

b) calculating the mean both ways for the following data on fines (in cents per day) for overdue books from medical libraries:

$$0, 0, 0, 0, 5, 5, 5, 5, 5, 5, 5, 10, 10, 10, 15, 25, 50.$$

5.2 The mean height of 30 boys and girls is given. Under what circumstances is this mean a legitimate summary statistic? Under what circumstances is it not?

5.3 What is the effect of an outlier on a mean? The mean annual payroll of all Maryland hospitals includes the annual payroll for Johns Hopkins Hospital. What would be the likely effect on the mean payroll figure if the value for Johns Hopkins Hospital was excluded?

5.4 Ten adult cadavers have heart diameters in millimeters as follows:

$$111, 125, 134, 119, 99, 123, 127, 120, 131, 122.$$

Find the mean, median, mode, range, and standard deviation.

5.5 Assume that the birth weights of infants are normally distributed with a mean weight of 8 lb and a standard deviation of 1 lb. Within which birth weights will 95% of all infants fall?

5.6 In a dental survey of pH of saliva, 2.5% of individuals were found to have a saliva pH greater than 8 and 2.5% had saliva with pH less than 6. Assuming a normal distribution, what is the mean and standard deviation of this distribution?

Table 5.2. Vital capacity measurements for 89 males aged 40 to 59 years (in liters)

5.15	4.57	6.16	3.89	4.81	4.57
5.89	5.17	4.48	4.48	5.89	6.84
4.27	5.20	4.16	5.22	4.59	3.80
3.69	6.37	3.91	5.71	5.31	4.48
3.80	3.37	5.20	5.04	4.90	5.80
4.84	5.49	4.75	4.72	4.43	3.60
4.00	3.28	4.57	4.59	3.35	4.18
4.54	4.14	4.18	3.64	5.38	4.66
3.46	3.44	5.62	5.96	5.74	5.26
4.39	4.86	5.38	6.68	4.25	4.36
5.76	3.71	5.76	5.06	7.51[b]	3.91
5.29	4.32	2.88[a]	4.86	3.67	4.63
5.51	5.49	6.14	5.22	4.59	6.13
3.56	4.66	5.51	5.51	4.18	5.87
5.02	4.61	4.57	4.27	4.43	

[a] Minimum.
[b] Maximum.

5.7 Table 5.2 gives vital capacity measurements for 89 males aged 40 to 59 years. Construct a frequency histogram for this data. From the histogram tell what proportion of the 89 males has a vital capacity less than or equal to 3.99 liters.

5.8 The Hospitals Administration Services Program gives the normal range of values for nursing (direct cost per patient per day) as from $20.90 to $33.40 for all participating hospitals with from 200 to 299 beds. The median is given as $25.93. Is there any evidence from this information that the distribution of nursing costs is asymmetrical?

5.9 Based on a sample of 50 years, the mean crude death rate is 13 per 1,000. If a standard deviation were given at the same time, what would it describe? Explain the difference between a histogram of crude death rates for 50 years and the usual graph showing the crude death rate each year.

LITERATURE CITED

Halperin, M., H. O. Hartley and P. G. Hoel. 1965. Recommended Standards for Statistical Symbols and Notation. Amer. Statis. 19(3):12.

6

Elementary Probability

6.1 INTRODUCTION

The concept of probability is fundamental to statistics. Two ideas are basic to the concept of probability. One is that probability is a measure of one's belief in the future occurrence of a specific event, such as becoming a parent within a year. The other is that probability measures the frequency with which an event such as pregnancy may occur in a long series of repeated trials, such as intercourse without contraception. For our purpose these two approaches to probability are considered as different aspects of one idea. This enables us to calculate a **probability** as a relative frequency, and also to consider it as a measure of belief held by the average person.

The conventional definition of probability in terms of frequency follows from considerations of identical repeated trials, each with the same number of mutually exclusive, exhaustive, and equally likely outcomes. Probability is then the frequency with which a given event occurs in these trials. Thus, if out of 200 sets of live-born twins delivered in a given period in a given area, 63 sets consisted of males only, the probability that both twins were male would be calculated as 63/200 or 31.5% or 0.315. Then if a pregnant woman was diagnosed as carrying twin embryos the probability of her twins both being boys would be 31.5% or 0.315.

It is implicit in this frequency definition that probability is measured on a scale ranging from 0 to 1 (or from 0% to 100%). A probability of 0 denotes an event which does not occur at all in the series of trials and is therefore considered to be an impossible event. Since on no day did the sun fail to rise, the probability that the sun will fail to rise tomorrow is 0. We can express this more simply by stating that the rising of the sun on any given day has a probability of 1, or certainty. It is conventional to measure probabilities on a decimal or percentage scale between 0 and 1 (or 0% to 100%). It is better to give the probability of, say, a child being born with a cleft lip or palate as 0.00125 or 0.125% or 1.25 per 1,000 or 12.5 per 10,000 than to say that 1 out of 800 children will exhibit this trait.

For the same reason probabilities are preferred to odds. Odds may be defined as the ratio of the frequency with which an event occurs, or is believed to occur, to the frequency with which it does not occur, or is believed not to occur. Thus, the odds that a patient will pay his bill in full before one month following discharge may be 3 : 1 (read 3 to 1). The equivalent probability is calculated from the odds by dividing the numerator of the odds by the sum of the numerator and denominator. Thus, odds of 3 : 1 are equivalent to a probability of 0.75 (3/4). Not only is it easier to make comparisons with probabilities than with odds, but probabilities may more readily be combined to calculate the probability of complex events.

Example. A study of adults reveals that the odds of being edentulous (without teeth) varies with the person's age. This information is given in Table 6.1 in terms of odds and probabilities. The

Table 6.1. Odds that an adult is edentulous by a specified age

Age (in years)	Odds	Probability
20–40	1 : 19	0.05
40–60	1 : 14	0.07
60–80	1 : 1	0.50

Amended from *Decayed, Missing and Filled Teeth in Adults, United States, 1960–1962.* National Center for Health Statistics, U.S. Department of Health, Education, and Welfare, Public Health Service Publication No. 1000, Ser. 11, No. 23.

probabilities in Table 6.1 can be compared as easily as their corresponding odds and they both show the increasing chance of a person's becoming edentulous as he grows older.

The following is an example in which odds are less easily compared.

Example. A physician knows that the odds of his being able to find a bed for a patient in each of three hospitals, A, B, C, are 3 : 5, 1 : 2, and 7 : 11, respectively. To decide which hospital he should call first, he needs to know which hospital has the highest probability of a vacant bed. These probabilities for the three hospitals are

$$A: \frac{3}{3+5} = \frac{3}{8} = 0.375 \text{ or } 37.5\%$$

$$B: \frac{1}{1+2} = \frac{1}{3} = 0.333 \text{ or } 33.3\%$$

$$C: \frac{7}{7+11} = \frac{7}{18} = 0.389 \text{ or } 38.9\%.$$

Clearly he should try the hospitals in the order C, A, B.

6.2 USES OF PROBABILITY

The main reason for introducing probability concepts is that they are basic to the concept of theoretical frequency distributions of statistical variables. As a result, statistical tests are stated in terms of probability. Also, as in the simple example above, probabilities can be used to evaluate the various outcomes of alternative decisions. Of course, there are other uses of probability, but the above uses are of most concern to us and will be exemplified in the following paragraphs.

From a knowledge of the appropriate distribution, we can calculate the probability that a continuous variable (or measure) falls between two specified values. We can also calculate the probability that a variable or statistic falls above or below a given specified value. These statements are generally written $P(c_1 < x \leqslant c_2)$, i.e., the probability that a continuous variable x will fall between constant values c_1 and c_2, and $P(x > c_1)$ or $P(x \leqslant c_2)$, i.e., the probability that a continuous variable x has a value above c_1 or below c_2. We use the theoretical distribution to calculate the probability that a discrete variable (or classification) takes on a certain value or falls in a given category or classification. For example, the probability that a newborn child is a boy is 51%. This is written $P(\text{boy}) = 0.51$ or $P(x = 0) = 0.51$, where $x = 0$ represents the event the child is a boy. Similarly, in a dental study the number of missing teeth is a discrete variable with integer values $0, 1, \ldots, 32$. We may represent the probability of being edentulous as $P(x = 32) = 0.18$. The probability of having a complete dentition is $P(x = 0) = 0.03$, and the probability of having more than six teeth missing is $P(x > 6) = 0.53$ (Kelly, Van Kirk, and Garst, 1967).

Reports of many research studies in medical care culminate in a test of **significance**, which is merely a statement of the probability that the observed difference between two groups has occurred by chance mechanisms. If the probability is low, traditionally below 5%, one can conclude that the observed difference is *not* the result of chance but is caused by the characteristics that differentiate the groups. The calculation of a test of significance depends on a knowledge of the sampling distribution of the test statistics. This is why a sound knowledge of probability concepts and theoretical frequency distributions is important in understanding statistical methods.

Decision theory is of more intuitive appeal to the non-research-minded administrator of health systems. As indicated, the probability used in decision theory is more appropriately considered as subjective. The probability of running out of a given medical supply can generally be forecast by the person responsible for maintaining that supply. Physicians and dentists work each day of their professional lives with subjective probabilities, since they are concerned with each patient's diagnosis and prognosis (Lusted, 1968). Probabilities thus enter naturally into the work of both the health professional and the health administrator, since all decisions are made (presumably) to minimize serious risks (side effects, fire hazards) while maximizing the chances of success and beneficial effects. Generally, the possible outcomes of a decision may be typified by the probability of their occurrence following a given decision and by a measure of their benefit or harm, or, in the case of a health administrator, by predicted costs or savings. Thus, both probabilities and costs are considered in the process of making a decision. This process occurs intuitively or subconsciously in the experienced administrator or physician. However, as more information becomes available through computerization of medical records and hospital bills, estimating probabilities and costs may be easier if the information is quantified. Chapter 10 illustrates these concepts further.

6.3 THE LAWS OF PROBABILITY

If two events are independent, then the probability that the two events occur is equal to the probability that one occurs times the probability that the other occurs and vice versa. For example, if the probability that both patient and doctor are late for the same appointment is equal to the probability that the patient is late times the probability that the doctor is late, these two events are independent. If, however, the patient has waited for the doctor in previous appointments, he may decide to be late, and thus minimize his likely waiting time. Similarly, the probability that an overdose is prescribed by a doctor may be independent of the probability of this being undetected by the nurse administering the treatment. The combined probability is then quite low, for if

$$P(\text{overdose prescribed}) = 0.03$$

and

$$P(\text{nurse fails to check the dose level}) = 0.20,$$

then, if these two events are independent,

$$
\begin{aligned}
P(\text{patient given overdose}) &= P(\text{overdose prescribed and not} \\
&\qquad \text{checked by nurse}) \\
&= P(\text{overdose prescribed}) \times P(\text{dose} \\
&\qquad \text{not checked by nurse}) \\
&= 0.03 \times 0.20 = 0.006 \text{ or 6 per } 1{,}000.
\end{aligned}
$$

However it is more likely that the nurse will screen all the prescriptions, taking special care to check drugs that are potentially dangerous and to check amounts prescribed that appear to be excessive. In other words, while probabilities of combined events may be calculated by multiplying their separate probabilities, the resultant probabilities are based on the assumption that the events are independent. Often, in the provision of health care, associated events are *not* independent, so that such estimated probabilities are misleading.

Even in situations where a physiological process suggests independence, it may not exist. For example, the sex of successive children is, as far as we can tell, independent, so that the probability that two successive children of the same parents are boys is (approximately) $0.5 \times 0.5 = 0.25$. However, many people maintain that some couples have a tendency to produce children of one sex rather than the other. Nevertheless, when the assumption of independence is valid, the system of checks and double checks or fail-safe mechanisms gives a low probability of error. In the same way the provision of a back-up generator for electricity in the operating room results in an extremely small probability of a total power failure during a surgical operation.

When two events are mutually exclusive (only one may occur), we add their individual probabilities to get the probability that either one or the other occurs. For instance, the event (at least one boy in a set of twins) is composed of two mutually exclusive

3% Name wrong   6% Bill wrong

0.5% Both wrong   8.5% Probability one or
                     the other or both wrong

Figure 6.1. Illustration of the derivation of the probability that a patient's bill will contain at least one of two errors.

events, (two boys) and (one boy and one girl). In the notation of probability this is

P(no. of boys > 0 in a set of twins)
$$= P(\text{no. of boys} = 1) + P(\text{no. of boys} = 2).$$

When events are not mutually exclusive, the probability that one or the other or both occur is calculated by adding the probabilities that each occurs and subtracting the probability that they occur together. For example, if 3% of patients' names are misspelled, 6% of their bills contain errors in arithmetic, and 0.5% contain both types of error, the probability that when any patient is discharged he will get a bill containing errors in either spelling of his name, the amount charged, or both, is $0.030 + 0.060 - 0.005 = 0.085$. The justification for subtracting the probability that both types of error occur is that otherwise we would be including that probability two times (see Figure 6.1).

6.4 CONDITIONAL PROBABILITIES

In health care, most events of interest affect one another; i.e., events are generally dependent on each other. When events are not independent, we can still calculate the probability of two events happening if we know the probability of one event occurring given that the other event has occurred. This is called **conditional probability**.

Examples. The probability that a pregnant woman is carrying twins is greater if she has had twins before or if her mother has had twins. This is expressed as follows:

$$P(\text{twins} \mid \text{twins before}) > P(\text{twins}).$$

The probability that a patient is unable to pay his bill is greater if he has a history of unpaid debts:

P(unable to pay bill | earlier record of unpaid bills)
$$> P(\text{unable to pay bill}).$$

The probability that a person dies of cancer of the lungs is higher if he is a heavy cigarette smoker:

P(death from lung cancer | cigarette smoker)
$$> P(\text{death from lung cancer}).$$

In general, if A and B are two events, then

$$P(AB) = P(A \mid B) \times P(B).$$

When A and B are independent,

$$P(AB) = P(A) \times P(B),$$

so that

$$P(A \mid B) = P(A)$$

Two events occur together more frequently when A and B are positively associated (e.g., if B predisposes toward A) and less frequently when A and B are negatively associated (e.g., when B inhibits the occurrence of A). This is directly analogous to the concept of correlation (see Section 9.7.1).

6.5   PRIOR INFORMATION AND BAYES' THEOREM

Consider the problem of the presence of the hepatitis virus in transfused blood. It is known that hepatitis is more likely to be present in blood taken from one who is a drug addict, in a low socioeconomic group, an urban resident, or institutionalized. Polissar (1969) shows how prior information may be used to increase the probability of detecting contaminated blood. Life insurance companies weight premiums using the fact that obesity is related to higher death rates. Automobile insurance companies likewise use prior information in deciding whether an applicant is a good risk, i.e., one with a low probability of accidents. The objective of preventive medicine and high risk registers is to detect those individuals at risk of future illnesses and to change their environment, habits, etc., thereby reducing their risks. Consider a highly artificial example in which a physician has observed a rash and an elevated temperature in a child and has narrowed down the possible causes to scarlet fever (SF), chicken pox (CP), and all other diseases (AOD). He knows from past experience that the incidence of these symptoms in cases of scarlet fever, chicken pox, and all other diseases is respectively 1, 0.85, 0.33. He also knows that in the community in which this child lives the incidence of these conditions is currently 5, 150, and 75 per 1,000. To convert these disease incidences into probabilities we divide each incidence by the sum of the incidence of disease. Thus the probability that the child has scarlet fever is

$$P(SF) = .005/(.005 + .150 + .075)$$
$$= .005/.230$$
$$= .022$$

Likewise

$$P(CP) = .150/.230$$
$$= .652$$

and

$$P(AOD) = .075/.230$$
$$= .326$$

(Note that $P(SF) + P(CP) + P(AOD) = 1.000$. However, as indicated in the next example we get the same result using the unconverted incidences of these three diseases in place of their probabilities.)

In symbolic notation,

$$P(\text{symptoms} \mid SF) = 1.00 \text{ where } P(SF) = .022$$
$$P(\text{symptoms} \mid CP) = 0.85 \text{ where } P(CP) = .652$$
$$P(\text{symptoms} \mid AOD) = 0.33 \text{ where } P(AOD) = .326$$

so that

$$P(\text{symptoms} \mid SF) \times P(SF) = 1.00 \times .022 = 0.022,$$
$$P(\text{symptoms} \mid CP) \times P(CP) = 0.85 \times .652 = 0.554,$$
$$P(\text{symptoms} \mid AOD) \times P(AOD) = 0.33 \times .326 = 0.108,$$
$$\text{Total} = 0.684.$$

We may now calculate the probability that the child has chicken pox, given that he has the observed symptoms, as follows:

$P(CP \mid \text{symptoms})$

$$= \frac{P(\text{symptoms} \mid CP) \times P(CP)}{P(\text{symptoms} \mid SF) \times P(SF) + P(\text{symptoms} \mid CP) \times P(CP) + P(\text{symptoms} \mid AOD) \times P(AOD)}$$

$$= \frac{0.554}{0.022 + 0.554 + 0.108} = \frac{0.554}{0.684} = 0.81 = 81\%.$$

Note that the high frequency of chicken pox in the community is influencing the calculation.

If S stands for symptoms or signs or other observations and A, B, C for the mutually exclusive and exhaustive set of diseases or events associated with S, we may state Bayes' theorem as

$$P(B \mid S) = \frac{P(S \mid B) \times P(B)}{P(S \mid A) \times P(A) + P(S \mid B) \times P(B) + P(S \mid C) \times P(C)}.$$

The calculation of $P(A \mid S)$ and $P(C \mid S)$ follows from similar expressions.

As another example, Bayes' theorem might be used in the determination of paternity. Assume that a child's blood group system is compatible with the blood groups of three possible fathers, X, Y, and Z. Then if $P(X)$, $P(Y)$, and $P(Z)$ represent the frequency of each man's blood group system in the population, and if $P(O \mid X)$, $P(O \mid Y)$, and $P(O \mid Z)$ are the probabilities of the offspring's blood group system given the mother's and a presumed father's blood group system, then we calculate

$$P(X \mid O) = \frac{P(O \mid X) \times P(X)}{P(O \mid X) \times P(X) + P(O \mid Y) \times P(Y) + P(O \mid Z) \times P(Z)}.$$

$P(Y \mid O)$ and $P(Z \mid O)$ are calculated similarly. The three men X, Y, and Z may then be ranked in order of their presumed paternity according to the relative magnitudes of $P(X \mid O)$, $P(Y \mid O)$, and $P(Z \mid O)$. Note that in this example $P(X)$, $P(Y)$, and $P(Z)$ do not necessarily add to 1. We could force this as in our first example on differential diagnosis by dividing each probability by their sum. This however, is unnecessary since the sum cancels in the expansion for Bayes' Theorem. The formula for $P(X \mid O)$ is therefore correct as given.

6.6   BINOMIAL PROBABILITIES

If there are only two possible outcomes in a given trial or event and $\mathcal{P}$ is the probability that one of these occurs and Q is the probability that the other occurs, then

$$Q = 1 - \mathcal{P}$$

Since $\mathcal{P} + Q = 1$. (There are only two mutually exclusive and exhaustive outcomes, so the sum of their probabilities is 1 or 100%.)

Example. Let S stand for success of a contraceptive in a given menstrual cycle and F for failure (i.e., pregnancy). Then if $\mathcal{P} = P(S)$ and $Q = P(F)$, the probability of success (i.e., no pregnancy after 12 months) is

$$\mathcal{P} \times \mathcal{P} \times \mathcal{P} \times \mathcal{P} \times \cdots \times \mathcal{P} = \mathcal{P}^{12}.$$

The probability of pregnancy in the third month is

$$\mathcal{P} \times \mathcal{P} \times Q = \mathcal{P}^2 Q.$$

In the above example it is meaningless to talk about a success in the month following a failure or to talk about two failures in succession. In general, however, the order of the probabilities is not important. For example, a family of two boys and one girl can be composed of, in the order of birth,

a boy, a boy, a girl;
a boy, a girl, a boy;
a girl, a boy, a boy.

If $\mathcal{P} = P(\text{boy})$ and $Q = P(\text{girl})$, then each of these three families will occur with a probability of $\mathcal{P}^2 Q$. It follows then that the probability of a two-boy and one-girl family, where the three children are born in any order, is $3\mathcal{P}^2 Q$. This term is a typical binomial probability and is represented generally by the formula

$$P(m \text{ successes in } n \text{ trials}) = \binom{n}{m} \mathcal{P}^m Q^{n-m}$$

where $\mathcal{P}$ and Q are defined as before, n is the number of repeated trials, m is the number of successes, and

$$\binom{n}{m} = \frac{n!}{m!(n-m)!}$$

gives the number of combinations of n things, m at a time (or the number of different ways in which m successes can occur among n trials).

The coefficients $\binom{n}{m}$ may also be generated by Pascal's triangle (see Exercise 6.3) or calculated from tables of factorials. As a result we may, for example, calculate the relative frequency of all possible ratios of boys to girls in families of six children, assuming that each child's sex is independent of the sexes of his or her siblings and that all mothers of six children have the same probability of giving birth to a boy first. The theoretical **binomial distribution**, then, is the relative frequency of all possible combinations derived from the laws of probability governing independent events (see Section 8.4).

EXERCISES

6.1 Two hospital indicators are considered to be independent. What is the probability that one will be above the upper **quartile** and the other below the median?

6.2 a) The probability that more than 6 teeth are decayed, missing, or filled is thought to be between 10% and 35%. Write this statement in symbols using standard notation.

    b) The probability that between 2 and 6 teeth are decayed, missing, or filled is given to be 0.53. Express this symbolically.

6.3 Pascal's triangle is a way of generating the binomial co-efficients $\binom{n}{m}$ by repeated addition. The triangle is built up row by row, each row corresponding to a value of n, the number of trials. The rule is to add each pair of adjacent values to give the value in the row.

n	values of $\binom{n}{m}$
0	1
1	1 1
2	1 2 1
3	1 3 3 1

To get the next line, add adjacent coefficients to get

4   1   4   6   4   1.

These values give the number of ways that 4 things can occur when 0, 1, 2, 3, or 4 are alike. Thus there are 6 ways in which 4 things can occur with 2 alike of one form (and 2 alike of the other form).

Let B and G stand for boy and girl, respectively. There are 6 ways in which a family of 4 with 2 boys and 2 girls can occur.

a) Enumerate these 6 different combinations.

b) Generate the next line of the triangle and state what each value stands for.

c) Five patients coded *U, V, W, X,* and *Y* are scheduled for an appointment at 9:00 A.M. Each is classified as early (*E*) or late (*L*). (None is on time.) Enumerate the possible combinations if 3 are late and 2 early.

6.4 A university hospital has a record of 130 "successful" kidney transplants out of 200. Other things being equal, what is the probability that the next kidney transplant in this hospital will be successful?

6.5 Eight percent of Black Americans are carriers of sickle cell anemia. A new test to detect the carrier gives a positive indication 97% of the time when the individual is a carrier and gives a negative indication 95% of the time when the individual is not a carrier. A Black American is selected at random from this population, is given the test, and reacts positively. What is the probability that he is a carrier? (Hint: Use Bayes' theorem.)

6.6 From past records it was discovered that 25% of all hospital bills contain an error or errors. A person is employed to check all bills before processing. The probability that he misclassifies a bill is 10%. What is the probability that if a bill is classified as correct it is actually correct? What is the probability that a bill which is classified as incorrect is in fact incorrect? (Hint: Use Bayes' theorem and assume he is as likely to misclassify a bill as incorrect when it is correct as to misclassify a bill as correct when it is incorrect.)

LITERATURE CITED

Kelly, J. E., L. E. Van Kirk and C. C. Garst, 1967. Decayed, Missing and Filled Teeth in Adults, U.S. 1960–62. N.C.H.S. Ser. 11, No. 23, U.S. Government Printing Office, Washington.

Lusted, L. B. 1968. Introduction to Medical Decision Making. Charles C Thomas, Springfield, Ill.

Polissar, J. 1969. Transfusion Hepatitis: Use of Statistical Decision Theory. Transfusion 9(1):15.

FURTHER READING

Gentleman, J. F. 1975. Generation of all $_NC_R$ combinations by nested Fortran *DO* loops. J. Roy. Statist. Soc. C (Appl. Statist.) 24(3):374–376.

Mathematical Thinking in Behavioral Sciences: Readings from Scientific American. Part I. The Analysis of Uncertainty: Probability. 1968. W. H. Freemen & Company, San Francisco.

7

Estimates and Confidence Limits
Use of Tables

7.1 INTRODUCTION

In this chapter we emphasize the concepts of estimation and
confidence limits and with the aid of tables demonstrate the use of
these concepts. A justification for the procedures used here, however, is deferred until the next chapter. Note that thus far we have
been concerned chiefly with descriptive statistics—how to reduce
statistical information to a few descriptive statistics such as the
mean and range. In this chapter and the ones that follow, we turn
to the more difficult but more rewarding topic of how to use
information from sample data to predict, within limits, the characteristics of the population. Once more we consider discrete and
continuous variables separately. Indeed let us begin by considering
the binomial variable which may take only two values, e.g., yes or
no, male or female, dead or alive, insured or uninsured.

7.2 ESTIMATES AND CONFIDENCE LIMITS FOR PROPORTIONS

As an illustration of the use of estimates and confidence limits,
consider a sample survey of the qualified nurses in a given hospital
or geographic area. Assume that the variable of interest is whether
a nurse received her professional training in the state or outside
the state in which she now works. We omit those who had both

Table 7.1. Feasible sample proportions by size of sample

Sample size	Fraction of nurses trained in-state: possible results					
1					0/1	1/1
2				0/2	1/2	2/2
3			0/3	1/3	2/3	3/3
4		0/4	1/4	2/4	3/4	4/4
.			.	.	.	.
.			.	.	.	.
.			.	.	.	.
n	0/n	1/n	. . .	m/n	. . .	n/n

in-state and out-of-state professional training on the grounds that these nurses do not fall into our population. A sample of size 1 (n = 1) has only two possible results: the nurse was trained either in-state or out-of-state. If a sample of two nurses is taken (n = 2), we can observe three possible results: both trained in-state, one trained in-state and one out-of-state, and both trained out-of-state. As the sample size increases we can tabulate all possible findings as in Table 7.1.

This table simply shows that for a binomial variable, a sample of size n can have 0, 1, 2, . . . , n sample units with the given characteristic. Therefore, a sample of size n has $n + 1$ possible outcomes (remember 0). If, in fact, we observe a sample of n units, with a number represented by m of the n having one characteristic (in-state training) and ($n - m$) the other characteristic (out-of-state training), we may call m/n the sample proportion p, so that $p = m/n$. For example, if 30 nurses are randomly selected and of these 23 have been trained in-state, then

$$p = m/n = 23/30 = 0.77 = 77\%.$$

Now in the total population (of trained nurses in the hospital or area) there is an overall proportion $\mathcal{P}$ with the characteristic (trained in-state). We could discover the value of $\mathcal{P}$, the population proportion, by taking a census and enumerating each member of the population. This might be possible in the population of nurses in a hospital but may not be practical for a large region such as a state. In any case, we may not want to know $\mathcal{P}$ to such a degree of accuracy that taking a census is justifiable. Therefore we take a random sample of size n and find that $p\%$ of these, i.e.,

$(m/n)\%$, have the characteristic (trained in-state). Theory shows that it is correct to follow our common sense and estimate the proportion in the population $\mathcal{P}$ by the proportion in the (random) sample p; i.e., if $p = 0.77$ in a sample of $n = 30$ nurses, then we estimate $\mathcal{P}$ to be 0.77 in the population of all nurses in the area. We can then state that from a sample survey, we estimate that 77% of all nurses have been trained in-state. We know, however, that this estimate of 77% is unlikely to be exactly the value of $\mathcal{P}$ in the population. Thus, a colleague who carries out an identical sample survey of the same population at the same time and uses the same sample size n will get her own estimate of $\mathcal{P}$, and her estimate will almost certainly differ from ours.

To indicate this variability, which is the result of sampling, it is common to report an estimate and its 95% confidence limits as well. These limits describe the range of estimates expected in 95 out of 100 repeated samples. Thus in our example $n = 30$ and $m = 23$, so that $p = 0.77$. From Table 7.2 we find that this lower limit is 57.72% and the upper limit is 90.07%.

A more complete description of these limits is that with 23 in-state trained nurses out of a sample of 30, we would be correct 95% of the time in asserting that the true proportion in the total population of nurses who were trained in-state was between 57.72% and 90.07%. This is written as

$$P(0.5772 \leqslant \mathcal{P} \leqslant 0.9007) = 0.95$$

or, in general,

$$P(p_l \leqslant \mathcal{P} \leqslant p_u) = \text{the size of the confidence level,}$$

where l is the lower limit and u the upper limit. (The difference between the two explanations of confidence limits is real, but numerically there is little difference between the two approaches. The reader should note that the second is the more generally accepted definition. However, if he finds the first more meaningful, he should use it since at this level he should not be led into error by its use.)

Example.   Of 24 successive blood donors, 6 were type O. Calculate the estimated proportion of type O individuals in the population, assuming the 24 blood donors to be a random sample with

Table 7.2. Exact 95% confidence limits for (P, given $p = m/n$, where n = sample size and m = number with the given characteristic

m	$p\%$	95% confidence limits
		$n = 2$
0	0.00	0.00- 84.19
1	50.00	1.26- 98.74
2	100.00	15.81-100.00
		$n = 3$
0	0.00	0.00- 70.76
1	33.33	0.84- 90.57
2	66.67	9.43- 99.16
3	100.00	29.24-100.00
		$n = 4$
0	0.00	0.00- 60.24
1	25.00	0.63- 80.59
2	50.00	6.76- 93.24
3	75.00	19.41- 99.37
4	100.00	39.76-100.00
		$n = 5$
0	0.00	0.00- 52.18
1	20.00	0.51- 71.64
2	40.00	5.27- 85.34
3	60.00	14.66- 94.73
4	80.00	28.36- 99.49
5	100.00	47.82-100.00
		$n = 6$
0	0.00	0.00- 45.93
1	16.67	0.42- 64.12
2	33.33	4.33- 77.72
3	50.00	11.81- 88.19
4	66.67	22.28- 95.67
5	83.33	35.88- 99.58
6	100.00	54.07-100.00
		$n = 7$
0	0.00	0.00- 40.96
1	14.29	0.36- 57.87
2	28.57	3.67- 70.96
3	42.86	9.90- 81.59
4	57.14	18.41- 90.10
5	71.43	29.04- 96.33
6	85.71	42.13- 99.64
7	100.00	59.04-100.00
		$n = 8$
0	0.00	0.00- 36.94
1	12.50	0.32- 52.65
2	25.00	3.19- 65.09
3	37.50	8.52- 75.51
4	50.00	15.70- 84.30
5	62.50	24.49- 91.48
6	75.00	34.91- 96.81
7	87.50	47.35- 99.68
8	100.00	63.06-100.00
		$n = 9$
0	0.00	0.00- 33.63
1	11.11	0.28- 48.25
2	22.22	2.81- 60.01
3	33.33	7.49- 70.07
4	44.44	13.70- 78.80
5	55.56	21.20- 86.30
6	66.67	29.93- 92.51
7	77.78	39.99- 97.19
8	88.89	51.75- 99.72
9	100.00	66.37-100.00
		$n = 10$
0	0.00	0.00- 30.85
1	10.00	0.25- 44.50
2	20.00	2.52- 55.61
3	30.00	6.67- 65.25
4	40.00	12.16- 73.76
5	50.00	18.71- 81.29
6	60.00	26.24- 87.84
7	70.00	34.75- 93.33
8	80.00	44.39- 97.48
9	90.00	55.50- 99.75
10	100.00	69.15-100.00
		$n = 11$
0	0.00	0.00- 28.49
1	9.09	0.23- 41.28
2	18.18	2.28- 51.78
3	27.27	6.02- 60.97
4	36.36	10.93- 69.21
5	45.45	16.75- 76.62
6	54.55	23.38- 83.25
7	63.64	30.79- 89.07
8	72.73	39.03- 93.98
9	81.82	48.22- 97.72

m	$p\%$	95% confidence limits
		$n = 11$ (continued)
10	90.91	58.72- 99.77
11	100.00	71.51-100.00
		$n = 12$
0	0.00	0.00- 26.46
1	8.33	0.21- 38.48
2	16.67	2.09- 48.41
3	25.00	5.49- 57.19
4	33.33	9.92- 65.11
5	41.67	15.17- 72.33
6	50.00	21.09- 78.91
7	58.33	27.67- 84.83
8	66.67	34.89- 90.08
9	75.00	42.81- 94.51
10	83.33	51.59- 97.91
11	91.67	61.52- 99.79
12	100.00	73.54-100.00
		$n = 13$
0	0.00	0.00- 24.71
1	7.69	0.19- 36.03
2	15.38	1.92- 45.45
3	23.08	5.04- 53.81
4	30.77	9.09- 61.43
5	38.46	13.86- 68.42
6	46.15	19.22- 74.87
7	53.85	25.13- 80.78
8	61.54	31.58- 86.14
9	69.23	38.57- 90.91
10	76.92	46.19- 94.96
11	84.62	54.55- 98.08
12	92.31	63.97- 99.81
13	100.00	75.29-100.00
		$n = 14$
0	0.00	0.00- 23.16
1	7.14	0.18- 33.87
2	14.29	1.78- 42.81
3	21.43	4.66- 50.80
4	28.57	8.39- 58.10
5	35.71	12.76- 64.86
6	42.86	17.66- 71.14
7	50.00	23.04- 76.96
8	57.14	28.86- 82.34
9	64.29	35.14- 87.24
10	71.43	41.90- 91.61
11	78.57	49.20- 95.34
12	85.71	57.19- 98.22
13	92.86	66.13- 99.82
14	100.00	76.84-100.00
		$n = 15$
0	0.00	0.00- 21.80
1	6.67	0.17- 31.95
2	13.33	1.66- 40.46
3	20.00	4.33- 48.09
4	26.67	7.79- 55.10
5	33.33	11.82- 61.62
6	40.00	16.34- 67.71
7	46.67	21.27- 73.41
8	53.33	26.59- 78.73
9	60.00	32.29- 83.66
10	66.67	38.38- 88.18
11	73.33	44.90- 92.21
12	80.00	51.91- 95.67
13	86.67	59.54- 98.34
14	93.33	68.05- 99.83
15	100.00	78.20-100.00
		$n = 16$
0	0.00	0.00- 20.59
1	6.25	0.16- 30.23
2	12.50	1.55- 38.35
3	18.75	4.05- 45.65
4	25.00	7.27- 52.38
5	31.25	11.02- 58.66
6	37.50	15.20- 64.57
7	43.75	19.75- 70.12
8	50.00	24.65- 75.35
9	56.25	29.88- 80.25
10	62.50	35.43- 84.80
11	68.75	41.34- 88.98
12	75.00	47.62- 92.73
13	81.25	54.35- 95.95
14	87.50	61.65- 98.45
15	93.75	69.77- 99.84
16	100.00	79.41-100.00
		$n = 17$
0	0.00	0.00- 19.51
1	5.88	0.15- 28.69
2	11.76	1.46- 36.44
3	17.65	3.80- 43.43
4	23.53	6.81- 49.90

m	$p\%$	95% confidence limits
		$n = 17$ (continued)
5	29.41	10.31- 55.96
6	35.29	14.21- 61.67
7	41.18	18.44- 67.08
8	47.06	22.98- 72.19
9	52.94	27.81- 77.02
10	58.82	32.92- 81.56
11	64.71	38.33- 85.79
12	70.59	44.04- 89.69
13	76.47	50.10- 93.19
14	82.35	56.57- 96.20
15	88.24	63.56- 98.54
16	94.12	71.31- 99.85
17	100.00	80.49-100.00
		$n = 18$
0	0.00	0.00- 18.53
1	5.56	0.14- 27.29
2	11.11	1.38- 34.71
3	16.67	3.58- 41.42
4	22.22	6.41- 47.64
5	27.78	9.69- 53.48
6	33.33	13.34- 59.01
7	38.89	17.30- 64.25
8	44.44	21.53- 69.24
9	50.00	26.02- 73.98
10	55.56	30.76- 78.47
11	61.11	35.75- 82.70
12	66.67	40.99- 86.66
13	72.22	46.52- 90.31
14	77.78	52.36- 93.59
15	83.33	58.58- 96.42
16	88.89	65.29- 98.62
17	94.44	72.71- 99.86
18	100.00	81.47-100.00
		$n = 19$
0	0.00	0.00- 17.65
1	5.26	0.13- 26.03
2	10.53	1.30- 33.14
3	15.79	3.38- 39.58
4	21.05	6.05- 45.57
5	26.32	9.15- 51.20
6	31.58	12.58- 56.55
7	36.84	16.29- 61.64
8	42.11	20.25- 66.50
9	47.37	24.45- 71.14
10	52.63	28.86- 75.55
11	57.89	33.50- 79.75
12	63.16	38.36- 83.71
13	68.42	43.45- 87.42
14	73.68	48.80- 90.85
15	78.95	54.43- 93.95
16	84.21	60.42- 96.62
17	89.47	66.86- 98.70
18	94.74	73.97- 99.87
19	100.00	82.35-100.00
		$n = 20$
0	0.00	0.00- 16.84
1	5.00	0.13- 24.87
2	10.00	1.23- 31.70
3	15.00	3.21- 37.89
4	20.00	5.73- 43.66
5	25.00	8.66- 49.10
6	30.00	11.89- 54.28
7	35.00	15.39- 59.22
8	40.00	19.12- 63.95
9	45.00	23.06- 68.47
10	50.00	27.20- 72.80
11	55.00	31.53- 76.94
12	60.00	36.05- 80.88
13	65.00	40.78- 84.61
14	70.00	45.72- 88.11
15	75.00	50.90- 91.34
16	80.00	56.34- 94.27
17	85.00	62.11- 96.79
18	90.00	68.30- 98.77
19	95.00	75.13- 99.87
20	100.00	83.16-100.00
		$n = 21$
0	0.00	0.00- 16.11
1	4.76	0.12- 23.82
2	9.52	1.17- 30.38
3	14.29	3.05- 36.34
4	19.05	5.45- 41.91
5	23.81	8.22- 47.17
6	28.57	11.28- 52.18
7	33.33	14.59- 56.97
8	38.10	18.11- 61.56
9	42.86	21.82- 65.98
10	47.62	25.71- 70.22
11	52.38	29.78- 74.29
12	57.14	34.02- 78.18
13	61.90	38.44- 81.89
14	66.67	43.03- 85.41

Table 7.2 (*Continued*)

m	p%	95% confidence limits
		n = 21 (continued)
15	71.43	47.82- 88.72
16	76.19	52.83- 91.78
17	80.95	58.09- 94.55
18	85.71	63.66- 96.95
19	90.48	69.62- 98.83
20	95.24	76.18- 99.88
21	100.00	83.89-100.00
		n = 22
0	0.00	0.00- 15.44
1	4.55	0.12- 22.84
2	9.09	1.12- 29.16
3	13.64	2.91- 34.91
4	18.18	5.19- 40.28
5	22.73	7.82- 45.37
6	27.27	10.73- 50.22
7	31.82	13.86- 54.87
8	36.36	17.20- 59.34
9	40.91	20.71- 63.65
10	45.45	24.39- 67.79
11	50.00	28.22- 71.78
12	54.55	32.21- 75.61
13	59.09	36.35- 79.29
14	63.64	40.66- 82.80
15	68.18	45.13- 86.14
16	72.73	49.78- 89.27
17	77.27	54.63- 92.18
18	81.82	59.72- 94.81
19	86.36	65.09- 97.09
20	90.91	70.84- 98.88
21	95.45	77.16- 99.88
22	100.00	84.56-100.00
		n = 23
0	0.00	0.00- 14.82
1	4.35	0.11- 21.95
2	8.70	1.07- 28.04
3	13.04	2.78- 33.59
4	17.39	4.95- 38.78
5	21.74	7.46- 43.70
6	26.09	10.23- 48.41
7	30.43	13.21- 52.92
8	34.78	16.38- 57.27
9	39.13	19.71- 61.46
10	43.48	23.19- 65.51
11	47.83	26.82- 69.41
12	52.17	30.59- 73.18
13	56.52	34.49- 76.81
14	60.87	38.54- 80.29
15	65.22	42.73- 83.62
16	69.57	47.08- 86.79
17	73.91	51.59- 89.77
18	78.26	56.30- 92.54
19	82.61	61.22- 95.05
20	86.96	66.41- 97.22
21	91.30	71.96- 98.93
22	95.65	78.05- 99.89
23	100.00	85.18-100.00
		n = 24
0	0.00	0.00- 14.25
1	4.17	0.11- 21.12
2	8.33	1.03- 27.00
3	12.50	2.66- 32.36
4	16.67	4.74- 37.38
5	20.83	7.13- 42.15
6	25.00	9.77- 46.71
7	29.17	12.62- 51.09
8	33.33	15.63- 55.32
9	37.50	18.80- 59.41
10	41.67	22.11- 63.36
11	45.83	25.55- 67.18
12	50.00	29.12- 70.88
13	54.17	32.82- 74.45
14	58.33	36.64- 77.89
15	62.50	40.59- 81.20
16	66.67	44.68- 84.37
17	70.83	48.91- 87.38
18	75.00	53.29- 90.23
19	79.17	57.85- 92.87
20	83.33	62.62- 95.26
21	87.50	67.64- 97.34
22	91.67	73.00- 98.97
23	95.83	78.88- 99.89
24	100.00	85.75-100.00
		n = 25
0	0.00	0.00- 13.72
1	4.00	0.10- 20.35
2	8.00	0.98- 26.03
3	12.00	2.55- 31.22
4	16.00	4.54- 36.08
5	20.00	6.83- 40.70
6	24.00	9.36- 45.13
7	28.00	12.07- 49.39
8	32.00	14.95- 53.50

m	p%	95% confidence limits
		n = 25 (continued)
9	36.00	17.97- 57.48
10	40.00	21.13- 61.33
11	44.00	24.40- 65.07
12	48.00	27.80- 68.69
13	52.00	31.31- 72.20
14	56.00	34.93- 75.60
15	60.00	38.67- 78.87
16	64.00	42.52- 82.03
17	68.00	46.50- 85.05
18	72.00	50.61- 87.93
19	76.00	54.87- 90.64
20	80.00	59.30- 93.17
21	84.00	63.92- 95.46
22	88.00	68.78- 97.45
23	92.00	73.97- 99.02
24	96.00	79.65- 99.90
25	100.00	86.28-100.00
		n = 26
0	0.00	0.00- 13.23
1	3.85	0.10- 19.64
2	7.69	0.95- 25.13
3	11.54	2.45- 30.15
4	15.38	4.36- 34.87
5	19.23	6.55- 39.35
6	23.08	8.97- 43.65
7	26.92	11.57- 47.79
8	30.77	14.33- 51.79
9	34.62	17.21- 55.67
10	38.46	20.23- 59.43
11	42.31	23.35- 63.08
12	46.15	26.59- 66.63
13	50.00	29.93- 70.07
14	53.85	33.37- 73.41
15	57.69	36.92- 76.65
16	61.54	40.57- 79.77
17	65.38	44.33- 82.79
18	69.23	48.21- 85.67
19	73.08	52.21- 88.43
20	76.92	56.35- 91.03
21	80.77	60.65- 93.45
22	84.62	65.13- 95.64
23	88.46	69.85- 97.55
24	92.31	74.87- 99.05
25	96.15	80.36- 99.90
26	100.00	86.77-100.00
		n = 27
0	0.00	0.00- 12.77
1	3.70	0.09- 18.97
2	7.41	0.91- 24.29
3	11.11	2.35- 29.16
4	14.81	4.19- 33.73
5	18.52	6.30- 38.08
6	22.22	8.62- 42.26
7	25.93	11.11- 46.28
8	29.63	13.75- 50.18
9	33.33	16.52- 53.96
10	37.04	19.40- 57.63
11	40.74	22.39- 61.20
12	44.44	25.48- 64.67
13	48.15	28.67- 68.05
14	51.85	31.95- 71.33
15	55.56	35.33- 74.52
16	59.26	38.80- 77.61
17	62.96	42.37- 80.60
18	66.67	46.04- 83.48
19	70.37	49.82- 86.25
20	74.07	53.72- 88.89
21	77.78	57.74- 91.38
22	81.48	61.92- 93.70
23	85.19	66.27- 95.81
24	88.89	70.84- 97.65
25	92.59	75.71- 99.09
26	96.30	81.03- 99.91
27	100.00	87.23-100.00
		n = 28
0	0.00	0.00- 12.34
1	3.57	0.09- 18.35
2	7.14	0.88- 23.50
3	10.71	2.27- 28.23
4	14.29	4.03- 32.67
5	17.86	6.06- 36.89
6	21.43	8.30- 40.95
7	25.00	10.69- 44.87
8	28.57	13.22- 48.67
9	32.14	15.88- 52.35
10	35.71	18.64- 55.93
11	39.29	21.50- 59.42
12	42.86	24.46- 62.82
13	46.43	27.51- 66.13
14	50.00	30.65- 69.35
15	53.57	33.87- 72.49
16	57.14	37.18- 75.54
17	60.71	40.58- 78.50

m	p%	95% confidence limits
		n = 28 (continued)
18	64.29	44.07- 81.36
19	67.86	47.65- 84.12
20	71.43	51.33- 86.78
21	75.00	55.13- 89.31
22	78.57	59.05- 91.70
23	82.14	63.11- 93.94
24	85.71	67.33- 95.97
25	89.29	71.77- 97.73
26	92.86	76.50- 99.12
27	96.43	81.65- 99.91
28	100.00	87.66-100.00
		n = 29
0	0.00	0.00- 11.94
1	3.45	0.09- 17.76
2	6.90	0.85- 22.77
3	10.34	2.19- 27.35
4	13.79	3.89- 31.66
5	17.24	5.85- 35.77
6	20.69	7.99- 39.72
7	24.14	10.30- 43.54
8	27.59	12.73- 47.24
9	31.03	15.28- 50.83
10	34.48	17.94- 54.33
11	37.93	20.69- 57.74
12	41.38	23.52- 61.06
13	44.83	26.45- 64.31
14	48.28	29.45- 67.47
15	51.72	32.53- 70.55
16	55.17	35.69- 73.55
17	58.62	38.94- 76.48
18	62.07	42.26- 79.31
19	65.52	45.67- 82.06
20	68.97	49.17- 84.72
21	72.41	52.76- 87.27
22	75.86	56.46- 89.70
23	79.31	60.28- 92.01
24	82.76	64.23- 94.15
25	86.21	68.34- 96.11
26	89.66	72.65- 97.81
27	93.10	77.23- 99.15
28	96.55	82.24- 99.91
29	100.00	88.06-100.00
		n = 30
0	0.00	0.00- 11.57
1	3.33	0.08- 17.22
2	6.67	0.82- 22.07
3	10.00	2.11- 26.53
4	13.33	3.76- 30.72
5	16.67	5.64- 34.72
6	20.00	7.71- 38.57
7	23.33	9.93- 42.28
8	26.67	12.28- 45.89
9	30.00	14.73- 49.40
10	33.33	17.29- 52.81
11	36.67	19.93- 56.14
12	40.00	22.66- 59.40
13	43.33	25.46- 62.57
14	46.67	28.34- 65.67
15	50.00	31.30- 68.70
16	53.33	34.33- 71.66
17	56.67	37.43- 74.54
18	60.00	40.60- 77.34
19	63.33	43.86- 80.07
20	66.67	47.19- 82.71
21	70.00	50.60- 85.27
22	73.33	54.11- 87.72
23	76.67	57.72- 90.07
24	80.00	61.43- 92.29
25	83.33	65.28- 94.36
26	86.67	69.28- 96.24
27	90.00	73.47- 97.89
28	93.33	77.93- 99.18
29	96.67	82.78- 99.92
30	100.00	88.43-100.00
		n = 31
0	0.00	0.00- 11.22
1	3.23	0.08- 16.70
2	6.45	0.79- 21.42
3	9.68	2.04- 25.75
4	12.90	3.63- 29.83
5	16.13	5.45- 33.73
6	19.35	7.45- 37.47
7	22.58	9.59- 41.10
8	25.81	11.86- 44.61
9	29.03	14.22- 48.04
10	32.26	16.68- 51.37
11	35.48	19.23- 54.63
12	38.71	21.85- 57.81
13	41.94	24.55- 60.92
14	45.16	27.32- 63.97
15	48.39	30.15- 66.94
16	51.61	33.06- 69.85
17	54.84	36.03- 72.68

Adapted from *Documenta Geigy Scientific Tables*, 7th ed., 1971, pp. 85-86, by permission of the publishers Ciba-Geigy Ltd., Basel, Switzerland.

regard to blood type. Also, calculate the 95% confidence limits of your estimate.

Since

$$p = \frac{6}{24} = 0.25 = 25\%,$$

we estimate $\mathcal{P}$ to be 25%; i.e., we estimate that 25% of the population has type O blood. From Table 7.2 we see that 95% confidence limits are 9.77% to 46.71%; i.e., 95% confidence limits for the frequency of type O blood in the population are 9.8% and 46.7%.

Often tables giving confidence limits for a proportion also give 99% limits. These are defined in a similar manner to 95% confidence limits. In other words, 99% confidence limits are those limits for which the probability that $\mathcal{P}$ falls within them is 99%. So far we have been restricted to a consideration of 95% and 99% confidence limits. These are conventional and are usually tabulated. However, there is no reason—apart from the lack of tables— why other levels of confidence for sample proportions cannot be used. Note that the above development for confidence limits of a proportion is not easily extended to discrete variables with three or more categories, i.e., to trinomial or multinomial classifications.

7.2.1 Sample Size

An important but unconventional use of tables such as Table 7.2 is to determine what size sample to take in a survey. In the conventional use of these tables, we know n, the sample size, and p, the sample proportion, and look up the confidence limits for $\mathcal{P}$. In using the tables to get n, we must know p and the approximate size of the confidence limits.

Example. A hospital administrator suspects that 30% of all reusable face masks are, in fact, used only once. He wishes to estimate this proportion in his hospital with 95% confidence limits that could range from 10% to 50%, i.e., the confidence limits could be 40% apart. Approximately how many of the face masks drawn from supplies should he investigate? An inspection of Table 7.2 gives $n = 23$ for $p = 30.43\%$ and 95% confidence limits of

13.21% to 52.92%. Therefore, the administrator should select and tag about 23 face masks to see what proportion is reused.

It may be argued that the decision to use 23 face masks depends on our knowing what we are trying to find, i.e., the proportion of face masks which are disposed of after one use. In the absence of prior information, i.e., if the investigator has no idea of what proportion he is going to find, the wisest procedure is to assume that $p = 50\%$. For 95% confidence limits 40% apart, this means that the lower and upper limits will be 30% and 70%, respectively. From Table 7.2 we find that for $n = 28$, 95% confidence limits for 50% are 30.65% and 69.35%. Therefore, to insure that his limits are not more than 20%, the investigator should take a sample of 28 or more face masks.

7.3 ESTIMATES AND CONFIDENCE LIMITS
FOR CONTINUOUS VARIATES NORMALLY DISTRIBUTED

7.3.1 The Mean

When the sample of n observations is randomly drawn, the sample mean is used to estimate the population mean:

$$\bar{x} \to \mu.$$

Just as a sample may give many different possible values for the proportion with a given characteristic, so may each sample of size n yield many different possible values for $\bar{x}$ and hence for the estimated μ. A measure of this variation is given by calculating 95% confidence limits for μ. These are the limits between which μ will fall with probability equal to 95%, that is,

$$P(\text{lower limit} \leqslant \mu \leqslant \text{upper limit}) = 0.95.$$

In a sample drawn at random from a population in which x is distributed normally, we use the sample standard deviation (s) to calculate 95% confidence limits. These limits are defined as

$$\bar{x} \pm k \times s$$

where k is the coefficient given in Table 7.3 for the appropriate sample size n and confidence level.

Table 7.3. Value of the constant k to be used in the formula $\bar{x} \pm ks$ in calculating 95% confidence limits for the population mean μ from a sample of size n

n	0	1	2	3	4	5	6	7	8	9
0			8.9845	2.4842	1.5913	1.2416	1.0494	0.9248	0.8360	0.7687
10	0.7154	0.6718	0.6354	0.6043	0.5774	0.5538	0.5329	0.5142	0.4973	0.4820
20	0.4680	0.4552	0.4434	0.4324	0.4223	0.4128	0.4039	0.3956	0.3878	0.3804
30	0.3734	0.3668	0.3605	0.3546	0.3489	0.3435	0.3384	0.3334	0.3287	0.3242
40	0.3198	0.3156	0.3116	0.3078	0.3040	0.3004	0.2970	0.2936	0.2904	0.2872
50	0.2842	0.2813	0.2784	0.2756	0.2730	0.2703	0.2678	0.2653	0.2629	0.2606
60	0.2583	0.2561	0.2540	0.2519	0.2498	0.2478	0.2458	0.2439	0.2421	0.2402
70	0.2385	0.2367	0.2350	0.2333	0.2317	0.2301	0.2285	0.2270	0.2255	0.2240
80	0.2225	0.2211	0.2197	0.2184	0.2170	0.2157	0.2144	0.2131	0.2119	0.2107
90	0.2095	0.2083	0.2071	0.2060	0.2048	0.2037	0.2026	0.2016	0.2005	0.1995
100	0.1984	0.1974	0.1964	0.1954	0.1945	0.1935	0.1926	0.1917	0.1908	0.1899
110	0.1890	0.1881	0.1872	0.1864	0.1856	0.1847	0.1839	0.1831	0.1823	0.1815
120	0.1808	0.1800	0.1792	0.1785	0.1778	0.1770	0.1763	0.1756	0.1749	0.1742
130	0.1735	0.1729	0.1722	0.1715	0.1709	0.1702	0.1696	0.1690	0.1683	0.1677
140	0.1671	0.1665	0.1659	0.1653	0.1647	0.1642	0.1636	0.1630	0.1625	0.1619
150	0.1614	0.1608	0.1603	0.1597	0.1592	0.1587	0.1582	0.1577	0.1571	0.1566
160	0.1561	0.1556	0.1551	0.1547	0.1542	0.1537	0.1533	0.1528	0.1523	0.1519
170	0.1514	0.1510	0.1505	0.1501	0.1496	0.1492	0.1488	0.1483	0.1479	0.1475
180	0.1471	0.1467	0.1463	0.1459	0.1455	0.1451	0.1447	0.1443	0.1439	0.1435
190	0.1431	0.1427	0.1424	0.1420	0.1416	0.1412	0.1409	0.1405	0.1402	0.1398
200	0.1394	0.1391	0.1388	0.1384	0.1381	0.1378	0.1375	0.1372	0.1369	0.1366
210	0.1362	0.1359	0.1356	0.1353	0.1350	0.1347	0.1344	0.1341	0.1338	0.1335
220	0.1328	0.1326	0.1323	0.1320	0.1317	0.1315	0.1313	0.1310	0.1308	0.1306
230	0.1372	0.1376	0.1379	0.1343	0.1340	0.1337	0.1334	0.1331	0.1328	0.1324
240	0.1255	0.1263	0.1260	0.1257	0.1255	0.1252	0.1250	0.1247	0.1245	0.1242
250	0.1240	0.1237	0.1235	0.1232	0.1230	0.1227	0.1225	0.1223	0.1220	0.1218
260	0.1216	0.1213	0.1211	0.1209	0.1206	0.1204	0.1202	0.1200	0.1197	0.1195
270	0.1193	0.1191	0.1188	0.1186	0.1184	0.1182	0.1180	0.1178	0.1176	0.1173
280	0.1171	0.1169	0.1167	0.1165	0.1163	0.1161	0.1159	0.1157	0.1155	0.1153
290	0.1151	0.1149	0.1147	0.1145	0.1143	0.1141	0.1139	0.1137	0.1135	0.1134
300	0.1132	0.1130	0.1128	0.1126	0.1124	0.1122	0.1120	0.1119	0.1117	0.1115
310	0.1113	0.1111	0.1110	0.1108	0.1106	0.1104	0.1103	0.1101	0.1099	0.1097
320	0.1096	0.1094	0.1092	0.1091	0.1089	0.1087	0.1086	0.1084	0.1082	0.1081
330	0.1079	0.1077	0.1076	0.1074	0.1072	0.1071	0.1069	0.1068	0.1066	0.1065
340	0.1063	0.1061	0.1060	0.1058	0.1057	0.1055	0.1054	0.1052	0.1051	0.1049
350	0.1048	0.1046	0.1045	0.1043	0.1042	0.1040	0.1039	0.1037	0.1036	0.1034
360	0.1033	0.1032	0.1030	0.1029	0.1027	0.1026	0.1025	0.1023	0.1022	0.1020
370	0.1019	0.1018	0.1016	0.1015	0.1014	0.1012	0.1011	0.1009	0.1008	0.1007
380	0.1005	0.1004	0.1003	0.1002	0.1000	0.0999	0.0998	0.0996	0.0995	0.0994
390	0.0993	0.0991	0.0990	0.0989	0.0988	0.0986	0.0985	0.0984	0.0982	0.0981
400	0.0980	0.0979	0.0978	0.0976	0.0975	0.0974	0.0973	0.0972	0.0970	0.0969
410	0.0968	0.0967	0.0966	0.0964	0.0963	0.0962	0.0961	0.0960	0.0959	0.0958
420	0.0956	0.0955	0.0954	0.0953	0.0952	0.0951	0.0950	0.0949	0.0947	0.0946
430	0.0945	0.0944	0.0943	0.0942	0.0941	0.0940	0.0939	0.0938	0.0937	0.0935
440	0.0934	0.0933	0.0932	0.0931	0.0930	0.0929	0.0928	0.0927	0.0926	0.0925
450	0.0924	0.0923	0.0922	0.0921	0.0920	0.0919	0.0918	0.0917	0.0916	0.0915
460	0.0914	0.0913	0.0912	0.0911	0.0910	0.0909	0.0908	0.0907	0.0906	0.0905
470	0.0904	0.0903	0.0902	0.0901	0.0900	0.0899	0.0898	0.0897	0.0896	0.0895
480	0.0894	0.0893	0.0892	0.0891	0.0890	0.0889	0.0888	0.0887	0.0887	0.0886
490	0.0885	0.0884	0.0884	0.0883	0.0882	0.0881	0.0880	0.0879	0.0878	0.0877

n	0	1	2	3	4	5	6	7	8	9
500	0.0877	0.0876	0.0875	0.0874	0.0873	0.0872	0.0871	0.0871	0.0870	0.0869
510	0.0868	0.0867	0.0866	0.0865	0.0865	0.0864	0.0863	0.0862	0.0861	0.0860
520	0.0860	0.0859	0.0858	0.0857	0.0856	0.0855	0.0854	0.0854	0.0853	0.0852
530	0.0851	0.0851	0.0850	0.0849	0.0848	0.0847	0.0847	0.0846	0.0845	0.0844
540	0.0843	0.0843	0.0842	0.0841	0.0840	0.0840	0.0839	0.0838	0.0837	0.0837
550	0.0836	0.0835	0.0834	0.0834	0.0833	0.0832	0.0831	0.0831	0.0830	0.0829
560	0.0828	0.0827	0.0826	0.0826	0.0825	0.0825	0.0824	0.0823	0.0822	0.0822
570	0.0821	0.0820	0.0819	0.0819	0.0818	0.0817	0.0817	0.0816	0.0815	0.0815
580	0.0814	0.0813	0.0812	0.0812	0.0811	0.0810	0.0810	0.0809	0.0808	0.0808
590	0.0807	0.0806	0.0806	0.0805	0.0804	0.0804	0.0803	0.0802	0.0802	0.0801
600	0.0800	0.0800	0.0799	0.0798	0.0798	0.0797	0.0796	0.0796	0.0795	0.0794
610	0.0794	0.0793	0.0793	0.0792	0.0791	0.0790	0.0790	0.0789	0.0788	0.0788
620	0.0787	0.0786	0.0786	0.0785	0.0785	0.0784	0.0783	0.0783	0.0782	0.0782
630	0.0781	0.0780	0.0780	0.0779	0.0779	0.0778	0.0777	0.0777	0.0776	0.0775
640	0.0775	0.0774	0.0773	0.0773	0.0772	0.0772	0.0771	0.0771	0.0770	0.0769
650	0.0769	0.0768	0.0767	0.0767	0.0766	0.0766	0.0765	0.0765	0.0764	0.0764
660	0.0763	0.0762	0.0762	0.0761	0.0761	0.0760	0.0760	0.0759	0.0758	0.0758
670	0.0757	0.0757	0.0756	0.0756	0.0755	0.0755	0.0754	0.0753	0.0753	0.0752
680	0.0752	0.0751	0.0751	0.0750	0.0750	0.0749	0.0748	0.0748	0.0747	0.0747
690	0.0746	0.0746	0.0745	0.0745	0.0744	0.0743	0.0743	0.0742	0.0742	0.0741
700	0.0741	0.0740	0.0740	0.0739	0.0739	0.0738	0.0738	0.0737	0.0737	0.0736
710	0.0736	0.0735	0.0735	0.0734	0.0734	0.0733	0.0733	0.0732	0.0732	0.0731
720	0.0731	0.0730	0.0729	0.0729	0.0728	0.0728	0.0727	0.0727	0.0726	0.0726
730	0.0726	0.0725	0.0725	0.0724	0.0724	0.0723	0.0723	0.0722	0.0722	0.0721
740	0.0721	0.0720	0.0720	0.0719	0.0719	0.0719	0.0718	0.0718	0.0717	0.0717
750	0.0716	0.0716	0.0716	0.0715	0.0715	0.0714	0.0714	0.0713	0.0713	0.0712
760	0.0712	0.0712	0.0711	0.0711	0.0710	0.0710	0.0709	0.0709	0.0708	0.0708
770	0.0707	0.0707	0.0706	0.0706	0.0705	0.0705	0.0705	0.0704	0.0704	0.0703
780	0.0703	0.0702	0.0702	0.0701	0.0701	0.0701	0.0700	0.0700	0.0699	0.0699
790	0.0698	0.0698	0.0698	0.0697	0.0697	0.0696	0.0696	0.0695	0.0695	0.0694
800	0.0693	0.0693	0.0692	0.0692	0.0691	0.0691	0.0690	0.0690	0.0690	0.0689
810	0.0689	0.0688	0.0688	0.0688	0.0687	0.0687	0.0686	0.0686	0.0685	0.0685
820	0.0684	0.0684	0.0684	0.0683	0.0683	0.0682	0.0682	0.0681	0.0681	0.0681
830	0.0680	0.0680	0.0679	0.0679	0.0679	0.0678	0.0678	0.0677	0.0677	0.0677
840	0.0676	0.0676	0.0675	0.0675	0.0674	0.0674	0.0674	0.0673	0.0673	0.0672
850	0.0672	0.0671	0.0671	0.0671	0.0670	0.0670	0.0669	0.0669	0.0669	0.0668
860	0.0668	0.0667	0.0667	0.0666	0.0666	0.0665	0.0665	0.0665	0.0664	0.0664
870	0.0663	0.0663	0.0662	0.0662	0.0662	0.0661	0.0661	0.0660	0.0660	0.0660
880	0.0659	0.0659	0.0658	0.0658	0.0658	0.0657	0.0657	0.0656	0.0656	0.0656
890	0.0655	0.0655	0.0654	0.0654	0.0654	0.0653	0.0653	0.0653	0.0652	0.0652
900	0.0650	0.0650	0.0649	0.0649	0.0649	0.0648	0.0648	0.0648	0.0647	0.0647
910	0.0647	0.0646	0.0646	0.0646	0.0645	0.0645	0.0645	0.0644	0.0644	0.0644
920	0.0643	0.0643	0.0642	0.0642	0.0642	0.0641	0.0641	0.0641	0.0640	0.0640
930	0.0639	0.0639	0.0639	0.0638	0.0638	0.0638	0.0637	0.0637	0.0637	0.0636
940	0.0639	0.0639	0.0638	0.0635	0.0635	0.0635	0.0634	0.0634	0.0634	0.0633
950	0.0636	0.0632	0.0632	0.0631	0.0631	0.0631	0.0630	0.0630	0.0630	0.0633
960	0.0633	0.0632	0.0629	0.0629	0.0628	0.0628	0.0628	0.0627	0.0630	0.0630
970	0.0629	0.0626	0.0626	0.0626	0.0625	0.0631	0.0628	0.0628	0.0627	0.0627
980	0.0623	0.0623	0.0625	0.0629	0.0626	0.0625	0.0624	0.0624	0.0623	0.0623
990	0.0620	0.0623	0.0626	0.0622	0.0622	0.0621	0.0621	0.0620	0.0620	0.0620
1000	0.0620									

From *Documenta Geigy Scientific Tables*, 7th ed., 1971, p. 43, by permission of the publishers Ciba-Geigy Ltd., Basel, Switzerland.

Example.   In 135 primipara, the duration of labor had a mean of 7 hr 35 min ($\bar{x}$) with a standard deviation of 48 min (s). Calculate the 95% confidence limits for the estimated mean duration of labor in all primipara, assuming that these 135 durations are a random sample of all primipara labor durations.

From Table 7.3, we find that

k, for $n = 135$ and 95% confidence limits, is 0.1702.

The 95% confidence limits for the unknown mean duration of labor, therefore, are

7 hr 35 min ± 0.1702 × 48 min = 7 hr 35 min ± 8.2 min;

i.e., the 95% confidence limits for the mean duration of labor of primipara are from 7 hr 26.8 min to 7 hr 43.2 min.

Often the confidence limits for a population mean are wrongly interpreted as the limits within which 95% of the population of x-values falls with 95% confidence. The two concepts are quite different, the **tolerance limits** within which 95% of the population falls being for all samples $n > 2$, much wider than the confidence limits for the mean. Thus, in the above example, for first babies, 95% of all durations of labor should, with 95% confidence, fall within

7 hr 35 min ± 2.19 × 48 min,
7 hr 35 min ± 105 min,
7 hr 35 min ± 1 hr 40 min,

i.e., from 5 hr 55 min to 9 hr 15 min. (The value 2.19 used to calculate these tolerance limits is derived from published tables of such coefficients; see, for example, *Documenta Geigy Scientific Tables.*)

We can use confidence limit tables to derive the appropriate sample size required to give limits a given distance apart, assuming that the standard deviation is known fairly well.

Example.   In the above example on the mean duration of labor, assume that we want to know what size of sample to take to give 95% confidence limits of not more than 30 minutes apart. This means that

$k \times s = 15$ min   so that $k = 15/s$.

Now if s is thought to be of the order of 50 min, then

$$k = 15/50 = 0.30.$$

Reading Table 7.3 (backward) gives $n = 45$ for a k-value of 0.30 for 95% confidence limits.

7.3.2 The Standard Deviation

Generally, one calculates the mean and standard deviation in a random sample of a continuous variable x drawn from a population that is normally distributed. We have shown how we estimate the population mean and its confidence limits. We may also estimate the population standard deviation and its confidence limits from a knowledge of the sample standard deviation.

Example. Assume that in a sample of 15 observations on water specimens, the fluoride content had a variation measured by a standard deviation of 3.3 ppm. From Table 7.4, using $n = 15$, we estimate the standard deviation of all replicate readings of fluoride from this water source to be

$$1.0180 \times 3.3 \text{ ppm} = 3.36$$

with 95% confidence limits

$$\text{from } 0.7321 \times 3.3 \text{ ppm} = 2.416$$
$$\text{to } \quad 1.577 \quad \times 3.3 \text{ ppm} = 5.204.$$

Table 7.4 can also be used to calculate the sample size required to estimate the population standard deviation within certain specified 95% confidence limits, though this figure is not often required.

Example. Assume that we want to estimate the population standard deviation to within ± 20% of the estimate; i.e., 95% confidence limits of σ should be approximately 0.80σ and 1.20σ. Examining Table 7.4, we see that for 95% confidence, $n = 53$ gives 0.8394 and 1.237, a range of just less than 40%. (Note that the confidence limits are *not* symmetrical about σ.)

7.4 DISTRIBUTION-FREE STATISTICS

The above tables are based on the population of the normal distribution of a continuous variable x. In situations where x is

Table 7.4. Correction factor k for an unbiased estimate of σ and 95% confidence limits of σ calculated from the standard deviation for a sample of size n

n	k	95% confidence limits
2	1.2533	0.4463-31.910
3	1.1284	0.5207- 6.285
4	1.0854	0.5665- 3.729
5	1.0638	0.5991- 2.874
6	1.0509	0.6242- 2.453
7	1.0424	0.6444- 2.202
8	1.0362	0.6612- 2.035
9	1.0317	0.6755- 1.916
10	1.0281	0.6878- 1.826
11	1.0253	0.6987- 1.755
12	1.0230	0.7084- 1.698
13	1.0210	0.7171- 1.651
14	1.0194	0.7250- 1.611
15	1.0180	0.7321- 1.577
16	1.0168	0.7387- 1.548
17	1.0157	0.7448- 1.522
18	1.0148	0.7504- 1.499
19	1.0140	0.7556- 1.479
20	1.0132	0.7604- 1.461
21	1.0126	0.7651- 1.444
22	1.0120	0.7694- 1.429
23	1.0114	0.7734- 1.415
24	1.0109	0.7772- 1.403
25	1.0105	0.7808- 1.391
26	1.0100	0.7843- 1.380
27	1.0097	0.7875- 1.370
28	1.0093	0.7906- 1.361
29	1.0090	0.7936- 1.352
30	1.0087	0.7964- 1.344
31	1.0084	0.7991- 1.337
32	1.0081	0.8017- 1.329
33	1.0078	0.8042- 1.323
34	1.0076	0.8066- 1.316
35	1.0074	0.8089- 1.310
36	1.0072	0.8111- 1.304
37	1.0070	0.8132- 1.299
38	1.0068	0.8153- 1.294
39	1.0066	0.8172- 1.289
40	1.0064	0.8192- 1.284
41	1.0063	0.8210- 1.279
42	1.0061	0.8228- 1.275
43	1.0060	0.8245- 1.271
44	1.0058	0.8262- 1.267
45	1.0057	0.8279- 1.263
46	1.0056	0.8294- 1.260
47	1.0055	0.8310- 1.256
48	1.0053	0.8325- 1.253
49	1.0052	0.8339- 1.249
50	1.0051	0.8353- 1.246
51	1.0050	0.8367- 1.243
52	1.0049	0.8380- 1.240

Continued.

Table 7.4. (*Continued*)

n	k	95% confidence limits
53	1.0048	0.8394- 1.237
54	1.0047	0.8406- 1.235
55	1.0046	0.8419- 1.232
56	1.0046	0.8431- 1.229
57	1.0045	0.8443- 1.227
58	1.0044	0.8454- 1.224
59	1.0043	0.8465- 1.222
60	1.0043	0.8476- 1.220
61	1.0042	0.8487- 1.217
62	1.0041	0.8498- 1.215
63	1.0040	0.8508- 1.213
64	1.0040	0.8518- 1.211
65	1.0039	0.8528- 1.209
66	1.0039	0.8537- 1.207
67	1.0038	0.8547- 1.205
68	1.0037	0.8556- 1.203
69	1.0037	0.8565- 1.202
70	1.0036	0.8574- 1.200
71	1.0036	0.8583- 1.198
72	1.0035	0.8591- 1.197
73	1.0035	0.8600- 1.195
74	1.0034	0.8608- 1.193
75	1.0034	0.8616- 1.192
76	1.0033	0.8624- 1.190
77	1.0033	0.8632- 1.189
78	1.0033	0.8640- 1.187
79	1.0032	0.8647- 1.186
80	1.0032	0.8655- 1.184
81	1.0031	0.8662- 1.183
82	1.0031	0.8669- 1.182
83	1.0031	0.8676- 1.180
84	1.0030	0.8683- 1.179
85	1.0030	0.8690- 1.178
86	1.0030	0.8696- 1.177
87	1.0029	0.8703- 1.175
88	1.0029	0.8709- 1.174
89	1.0029	0.8716- 1.173
90	1.0028	0.8722- 1.172
91	1.0028	0.8728- 1.171
92	1.0028	0.8734- 1.170
93	1.0027	0.8740- 1.169
94	1.0027	0.8746- 1.168
95	1.0027	0.8752- 1.167
96	1.0026	0.8758- 1.166
97	1.0026	0.8764- 1.165
98	1.0026	0.8769- 1.164
99	1.0026	0.8775- 1.163
100	1.0025	0.8780- 1.162

Amended from *Documenta Geigy Scientific Tables*, 7th ed., 1971, p. 47, by permission of the publishers Ciba-Geigy Ltd., Basel, Switzerland.

clearly not normally distributed we may use distribution-free confidence limits.

7.4.1 The Median

Example. The times at which automobile accidents occur follow a distribution that is certainly not normal. A sample of 33 accidents chosen at random has a median time of occurrence of 6:38 P.M. What are the 95% confidence limits of the population median μ_{50} from this sample of 33 accidents and the times they occurred?

The answer is obtained by consulting Table 7.5, which gives $x_{(11)}$ and $x_{(23)}$ as limits with a confidence level of 96.5%. (Because of the limited choice of ordered statistics to select, we cannot get exactly a 95% confidence limit.) Remember that $x_{(11)}$ is the eleventh smallest and $x_{(23)}$ the eleventh largest value in the sample.

Example. The duration of hospitalization for serious chronic conditions will not be normally distributed, especially if some patients die. Assume that nine patients with respiratory tuberculosis were hospitalized for 14, 16, 24, 36, 56, 60, 72, and 80 weeks and one patient died after 18 weeks. If we replace the death at 18 weeks by ∞, the median duration of 14, 16, 24, 36, 56, 60, 72, 80, and ∞ weeks is 56 weeks. Table 7.5 shows that for a sample of 9 the range between the second smallest and the second largest, i.e., from $x_{(2)}$ to $x_{(8)}$ or from 16 to 80 weeks, will give 96% confidence limits for the population median. (Note that in this example the mean of the sample is infinite. This is a situation in which, regardless of whether the distribution is normal or not, it is better to use the median rather than the mean.)

7.4.2 Tolerance Limits

Tolerance limits may be calculated irrespective of the form of the distribution. This distribution-free approach leads to Table 7.6, which gives the size of sample required to be $P\%$ confident that a given fraction (f) of the population lies between the smallest and largest observations in the sample.

Example. Fowler, Westcott, and Scott (1953) found that in 72 subjects the peak systolic pulmonary arterial blood pressure

Table 7.5. Confidence limits for the median lying between the ith smallest and largest observations in a sample of size n

n	i	Confidence level	n	i	Confidence level
3	1	0.750	20	4	0.997
4	1	.875		5	.988
5	1	.938		6	.959
6	1	.969		7	.885
	2	.781	21	5	.993
7	1	.984		6	.973
	2	.875		7	.922
8	1	.992		8	.811
	2	.930	22	5	.996
	3	.711		6	.983
9	1	.996		7	.948
	2	.961		8	.866
	3	.820	23	5	.997
10	1	.998		6	.989
	2	.979		7	.965
	3	.891		8	.907
11	1	.999		9	.790
	2	.988	24	6	.993
	3	.935		7	.977
	4	.773		8	.936
12	2	.994		9	.848
	3	.961	25	6	.996
	4	.854		7	.985
13	2	.997		8	.957
	3	.978		9	.892
	4	.908	26	7	.991
	5	.733		8	.971
14	2	.998		9	.924
	3	.987		10	.831
	4	.943	27	7	.994
	5	.820		8	.981
15	3	.993		9	.948
	4	.965		10	.878
	5	.882	28	7	.996
16	3	.996		8	.987
	4	.979		9	.964
	5	.923		10	.913
	6	.790		11	.815
17	3	.998	29	8	.992
	4	.987		9	.976
	5	.951		10	.939
	6	.857		11	.864
18	4	.992	30	8	.995
	5	.969		9	.984
	6	.904		10	.957
	7	.762		11	.901
19	4	.996		12	.800
	5	.981	31	8	.997
	6	.936		9	.989
	7	.833		10	.971

Table 7.5. (*Continued*)

n	i	Confidence level	n	i	Confidence level
31	11	0.929	41	15	0.940
	12	.850		16	.883
32	9	.993	42	13	.992
	10	.980		14	.980
	11	.950		15	.956
	12	.890		16	.912
33	9	.995		17	.836
	10	.986	43	13	.995
	11	.965		14	.986
	12	.920		15	.968
	13	.837		16	.934
34	10	.991		17	.874
	11	.976	44	14	.990
	12	.942		15	.977
	13	.879		16	.951
35	10	.994		17	.904
	11	.983		18	.826
	12	.959	45	14	.993
	13	.910		15	.984
	14	.825		16	.964
36	10	.996		17	.928
	11	.989		18	.865
	12	.971	46	14	.995
	13	.935		15	.989
	14	.868		16	.974
37	11	.992		17	.946
	12	.980		18	.896
	13	.953	47	15	.992
	14	.901		16	.981
	15	.812		17	.960
38	11	.995		18	.921
	12	.986		19	.856
	13	.966	48	15	.994
	14	.927		16	.987
	15	.857		17	.971
39	12	.991		18	.941
	13	.976		19	.889
	14	.947	49	16	.991
	15	.892		17	.979
40	12	.994		18	.956
	13	.983		19	.915
	14	.962		20	.848
	15	.919	50	16	.993
	16	.846		17	.985
41	12	.996		18	.967
	13	.988		19	.935
	14	.972		20	.881

From G. Noether, *Introduction to Statistics—A Fresh Approach,* Houghton Mifflin, Boston, 1971, p. 226, Table E.

Table 7.6. Minimum sample size required for a given fraction of the population (f) to lie within the sample range with a given level of confidence

Confidence level $(P\%)$	Fraction of the population lying between the lowest and highest values in the sample									
	0.999	0.99	0.95	0.90	0.80	0.70	0.60	0.50	0.40	0.30
99.9	9,230	919	181	88	42	27	19	14	11	9
99	6,636	661	130	64	31	20	14	10	8	6
98	5,832	581	115	56	27	17	12	9	7	6
95	4,742	473	93	45	22	14	10	7	6	5
90	3,889	388	77	38	18	12	8	6	5	4

Amended from *Documenta Geigy Scientific Tables*, 7th ed., 1971, p. 128, by permission of the publishers Ciba-Geigy Ltd., Basel, Switzerland.

ranged from 11 to 29 mm Hg. With what confidence can we state that 95% of the population will fall within this range?

Table 7.6 shows that the fraction 0.95 of the population will fall between the lowest and highest observations in a sample of 77 with a confidence level of 90%. There is, therefore, a confidence level just less than 90% that 95% of the population will have peak systolic blood pressures for the pulmonary artery between 11 and 29 mm Hg.

EXERCISES

7.1 At an AHA convention, 13 graduates of a program, who are now scattered throughout the US, compared notes on the daily cost per patient day at each of their respective hospitals. These are:

$86.25, 64.00, 73.20, 81.00, 82.40, 78.00
82.60, 74.25, 86.00, 69.90, 93.00, 82.40

and one known only to be over 90.00 per day. On the basis of this information, what are the 90% confidence limits for the average daily cost per patient assuming that the median is used?

7.2 A HMO launches an intensive campaign to increase the productivity of the health care professionals in the system. After one week, a random sample of 150 of the HMO employees is selected and their records examined. For each, an index of increased productivity is calculated. The mean and standard deviation of the 150 values of this index of increased productivity are 32 ± 40. Calculate the 95% confidence limits of the unknown mean. Describe this population mean in words. What conclusion with regard to the campaign do you draw? Note that a zero value is equivalent to no increase in productivity.

7.3 On a given day, the 30 medical beds in a given hospital were occupied by 5 blacks and 25 whites. An official visiting the hospital that day claimed that there appeared to be preferential treatment for whites. The hospital administrator refuted this allegation by pointing out that of the 23 employees serving these beds, 9 were black. Show that the 95% confidence limits of the proportion of blacks in the community served by this hospital from these two samples overlap, so that both proportions (5 out of 30 and 9 out of 23) could have arisen from the same population by (random) sampling variation.

7.4 Each couple's children can be considered a random sample of all the children they might have. How many children would a couple have to produce to determine with 95% confidence the intrinsic sex ratio of their (potential) offspring to within ± 20%? (Assume no multiple births.)

7.5 What sample size is needed to ensure 95% confidence limits of ± $5 for an unknown mean of fringe benefits (in equivalent dollars per annum) for registered nurses if the standard deviation is thought to be $35?

7.6 Why are 99% confidence limits for a proportion always larger than 95% confidence limits?

7.7 A sample of 29 hospitals reports their cost per patient-day. The mean of the 29 observations is $85.00 with a standard deviation of $5.00.

a) Calculate the 95% confidence limits for the mean cost per patient-day for all hospitals from which these 29 are chosen.

b) What percentage of all hospitals will have costs per patient-day falling between the maximum and minimum values observed in the sample? (Give the confidence level used also.)

c) Estimate the population standard deviation and give its 95% confidence limits.

d) In which of the above parts of this exercise is it necessary to assume
   i) that the sample was randomly selected?
   ii) that the observations were normally distributed?
   iii) that the observations were independent of each other?

LITERATURE CITED

Fowler, N. O., R. N. Westcott and R. C. Scott. 1953. Normal Pressure in the Right Heart and Pulmonary Artery. Amer. Heart J. 46:264.

8

The Underlying Distribution
of Statistics
from Repeated Samples

8.1 INTRODUCTION

In this chapter we present a justification for the formulas used in the previous chapter. This section of the book will therefore be more theoretical than the previous ones and may be omitted if desired. Following Section 8.3, we consider the concept of confidence limits in large samples based on a given theoretical distribution. The tables given in Chapter 7 are usually limited to sample sizes less than 100. For samples greater than this, we use a formula to calculate the confidence limits.

8.2 CONFIDENCE LIMITS FOR THE MEDIAN

Consider a population containing an infinite number of values of a continuous variable x. Note that this variable can follow any distribution, but assume that the median μ_{50} of the population is known. If an observation x is taken from the population at random, i.e., ($n = 1$), a sample of size one, then either

$$x \leqslant \mu_{50} \quad \text{or} \quad x > \mu_{50}.$$

In each case, by the definition of the median of a population, the probability is 0.5, i.e.,

$$P(x \leqslant \mu_{50}) = 0.5 = P(x > \mu_{50}).$$

Now consider a random sample of two observations x_1 and x_2 so that $n = 2$. Order the two observations and relabel them so that now $x_{(1)} \leqslant x_{(2)}$. Then one of three cases must occur:

(i) $\mu_{50} < x_{(1)} \leqslant x_{(2)}$,

(ii) $x_{(1)} < \mu_{50} < x_{(2)}$, or

(iii) $x_{(1)} \leqslant x_{(2)} \leqslant \mu_{50}$

The probabilities for these cases are, respectively, 0.25, 0.50, and 0.25. Thus

$$P(\text{i}) = P(\text{iii}) = 0.25,$$

since the probability of drawing two observations which are both below or both above the population median is $0.5 \times 0.5 = 0.25$. Since the three are exhaustive, i.e.,

$$P(\text{i}) + P(\text{ii}) + P(\text{iii}) = 1$$

it follows that $P(\text{ii}) = 0.5$. Note that case (ii) is a crude form of a confidence interval for the population median in a sample of size 2. In fact, we can say with 50% confidence that, if we take any two observations from a continuous distribution, the population median will lie between them. (Let us hope that the two values are not the same, which theoretically occurs with a zero probability for a continuous distribution with an infinite number of values!)

If the sample is of a size 4, we can again arrange the observations in increasing order and then call the observations $x_{(1)} \leqslant x_{(2)} \leqslant x_{(3)} \leqslant x_{(4)}$.

Let us calculate the probability that the median μ_{50} lies between the first and the fourth observations:

$$
\begin{aligned}
P(x_{(1)} < \mu_{50} < x_{(4)}) \quad &= 1 - P(x_{(1)} \cdots x_{(4)} \leqslant \mu_{50}) - P(\mu_{50} \leqslant x_{(1)} \cdots x_{(4)}) \\
&= 1 - \left(\frac{1}{2} \times \frac{1}{2} \times \frac{1}{2} \times \frac{1}{2}\right) - \left(\frac{1}{2} \times \frac{1}{2} \times \frac{1}{2} \times \frac{1}{2}\right) \\
&= 1 - 2\left(\frac{1}{2}\right)^4 \\
&= 1 - \left(\frac{1}{2}\right)^3 \\
&= 1 - 0.125 \\
&= 0.875.
\end{aligned}
$$

Table 8.1. Probability that the population median μ_{50} will fall between the smallest and largest observations in a sample of size n chosen randomly from a continuous distribution

n	$1 - (0.5)^{n-1}$
3	0.750
4	.875
5	.938
6	.969
7	.984
8	.992
9	.996
10	.998

We can generalize this to any sample size, and by a similar argument show that the confidence level that the population median falls between the smallest and largest observations in a sample of size n is $1 - (0.5)^{n-1}$. This is tabulated in Table 8.1 for sample size 3 through 10.

We can narrow these confidence limits by taking the limits (where possible) as the second smallest and the second largest values in the sample, the third smallest and third largest, etc., until we get confidence limits with a confidence level corresponding approximately to the level we want. Thus, for a sample of size $n = 10$ the confidence level associated with various confidence limits of different size are as shown in Table 8.2. Therefore, if we

Table 8.2. Confidence levels for the median μ_{50} associated with various confidence limits defined on the ranked observations in a sample of size 10

Confidence limits	Confidence level
$x_{(1)}$ to $x_{(10)}$	0.998
$x_{(2)}$ to $x_{(9)}$	.979
$x_{(3)}$ to $x_{(8)}$	.891
$x_{(4)}$ to $x_{(7)}$	.657
$x_{(5)}$ to $x_{(6)}$	.246

wanted 95% confidence limits for the population median we would be forced, in a sample of size 10, to choose the second smallest and second largest values as confidence limits. These give a confidence level of 97.9%, somewhat higher than what we wanted. If we were prepared to use a 90% confidence level we would select, in a sample of size 10, the third smallest and third largest values with a confidence level of 89.1%.

The confidence level associated with confidence limits of $x_{(r)}$ to $x_{(n-r+1)}$, where n is the size of the sample and $x_{(r)}$ is the rth smallest value in the sample, is derived by

$$P(x_{(r)} < \mu_{50} < x_{(n-r+1)}) = 1 - \left[1 + \binom{n}{1} + \binom{n}{2} + \cdots + \binom{n}{r-1} \right] (0.5)^{n-1}$$

$$= 1 - \sum_{i=0}^{r-1} \binom{n}{i} \times (0.5)^{n-i},$$

where (see Section 6.6 and Exercise 6.3)

$$\binom{n}{i} = \frac{n!}{i!\,(n-i)!} = \frac{n(n-1)(n-2)\cdots(n-i+1)}{1\cdot 2\cdot 3\cdots i}.$$

8.3 CONFIDENCE LIMITS FOR A PROPORTION

Here the response is a discrete classification in two groups, Yes or No, Male or Female, Dead or Alive. A sample of 10 may contain from 0 to 10 items with the given attribute; i.e., before we take the sample we know that the proportion in the sample is going to take *one* of 11 possible values:

$$0.0, 0.1, 0.2, 0.3, 0.4, 0.5, 0.6, 0.7, 0.8, 0.9, \text{ or } 1.0.$$

So that, trivially, we know that the proportion will lie between 0 and 1 with 100% confidence. Assume that, in fact, the sample contains 5 items with the given characteristic, i.e., $p = 0.5$. We realize however that the proportion $\mathcal{P}$ in the population need not be 0.5. Indeed it need not take one of the 11 possible values, but may take almost any value from 0 to 1, since, in a very large population of size N, alternative values of $\mathcal{P}$ can be as close as $1/N$. In the following discussion we treat $\mathcal{P}$ as continuous, i.e., as though it could take any value between 0 and 1, $0 < \mathcal{P} < 1$.

Although $\mathcal{P}$ is unknown we can write the expression for finding 5 positives in a sample of size 10 as

$$\binom{10}{5} \mathcal{P}^5 (1-\mathcal{P})^5.$$

Similarly, the probability of finding 6, 7, . . . out of 10 is

$$\binom{10}{6} \mathcal{P}^6 (1-\mathcal{P})^4, \qquad \binom{10}{7} \mathcal{P}^7 (1-\mathcal{P})^3, \qquad \text{etc.,}$$

so that the probability of finding 5 or more positives in a sample of size 10 will be

$$\binom{10}{5} \mathcal{P}^5 (1-\mathcal{P})^5 + \binom{10}{6} \mathcal{P}^6 (1-\mathcal{P})^4 + \binom{10}{7} \mathcal{P}^7 (1-\mathcal{P})^3$$

$$+ \binom{10}{8} \mathcal{P}^8 (1-\mathcal{P})^2 + \binom{10}{9} \mathcal{P}^9 (1-\mathcal{P}) + \binom{10}{10} \mathcal{P}^{10},$$

which can be written in a shorter form as

$$P(p \geqslant 0.5 \mid n = 10, \mathcal{P}) = \sum_{i=5}^{10} \binom{10}{i} \mathcal{P}^i (1-\mathcal{P})^{10-i}.$$

Next we pick a value of $\mathcal{P}$ which will make this expression equal to some value, say 2.5%. In the case of a sample of size 10, a value of $\mathcal{P}$ equal to 0.1871 gives a probability of 5 or more positives out of 10 equal to 2.5%, or

$$P(p \geqslant 0.5 \mid n = 10, \mathcal{P} = 0.1871)$$

$$= \sum_{i=5}^{10} \binom{10}{i} 0.1871^i \times 0.8129^{10-i} = 2.5\%.$$

$\mathcal{P} = 0.1871$ is then the lower confidence limit for an unknown population proportion (when a sample of size 10 contains 5 positives).

We now calculate the value of the upper confidence limit in a similar manner. Thus, the probability that a sample of size 10 contains 5 or less positives will be

$$P(p \leqslant 0.5 \mid n = 10, \mathcal{P}) = \sum_{i=0}^{5} \binom{10}{i} \mathcal{P}^i (1-\mathcal{P})^{10-i}.$$

If we set this probability equal to 2.5%, we find that the value of

(P which will fit this relationship is 0.8129. This is the upper limit of the exact confidence limits for an unknown population proportion (P.

We have now created two one-sided confidence limits for the unknown population proportion (P. Having, by our criterion, excluded values below 0.1871 and above 0.8129 as unlikely we indicate the interval between these as our confidence limit and assert that we are 95% confident that the true value of (P will fall between them. The converse of this statement is that in 5 out of 100 samples of size 10, each of which contains 5 positives, the true or population proportion will fall either below the lower limit of 0.1871 or above the upper limit of 0.8129.

The concept of 95% confidence limits is, of course, not restricted to samples of a given size with a given proportion. In general, in all applications of 95% confidence limits used to delimit the value of (P, we expect to be wrong about 5% of the time. If such a rate of error is unacceptable, we must use 99% confidence limits which are similarly defined and extensively tabulated, or we must choose and calculate our own confidence limits.

8.4 SAMPLING DISTRIBUTION OF A PROPORTION

We can now reveal that in Section 8.3 we have, in fact, been using the concept of a sampling distribution of a proportion. To recapitulate, we are working with a binomial variate that takes only two values, say 0 and 1. We have a large (or infinite) population of items, (P% of which have the given attribute (i.e., $x = 1$). Therefore, in samples of size 1 (i.e., selecting an item at random from the population) the probability that this item has the attribute is (P, and the probability that it does not is $(1 - (P))\%$. We may write this as

$$P(x = 1) = (P \quad \text{and} \quad P(x = 0) = 1 - (P.$$

If the sample size is greater than 1, say $n = 10$, then we have 10 independently selected items from the population, each of which either has the attribute or does not, with probabilities (P and $(1 - (P))$, respectively. However, we can summarize the information in the sample by a single statistic. This, of course, is p, the proportion in the sample with the attribute. We have seen that p must have *one* of the $(n + 1)$ values

$$0/n, \ 1/n, \ 2/n, \ 3/n, \ \ldots, \ (n - 1)/n, \ n/n.$$

Indeed, using the laws of probability, we can calculate the probability of each of the above proportions occurring in a random sample of size n from a population with $\mathcal{P}\%$ having the attribute. This is the binomial probability

$$P(p = \frac{m}{n} \ \Big| \ n, (\mathcal{P})) = \binom{n}{m} \ (\mathcal{P}^m \ (1 - (\mathcal{P})^{n-m}$$

and if we calculate these binomial probabilities for each possible value of $m = 0, 1, \ldots, n,$ we have the binomial distribution. This binomial distribution is a **sampling distribution** in that it gives the probabilities of different values of a statistic p occurring in a future sample of size n.

We can generate this sampling distribution empirically by taking *repeated* random samples of size n from a given binomial population, calculating the statistic p for each sample and tabulating the resultant frequencies. Thus, if we take 100 samples of size 10, we have 100 statistics (values of p) which we can group into the 11 possible values that p can take in samples of size 10. Thus, we might find the frequency table given in Table 8.3. This is

Table 8.3. Empirical sampling distribution of the proportion p in 100 randomly selected samples, each of size 10

p	f
0/10	0
1/10	2
2/10	4
3/10	5
4/10	23
5/10	15
6/10	30
7/10	12
8/10	7
9/10	1
10/10	1
Total	100

an empirical sampling distribution, as contrasted to a theoretical sampling distribution, in which the frequencies of different values of p are calculated from binomial probabilities. Note, however, that we seldom if ever need to take multiple samples. Usually, in spite of the emphasis in this section on repeated sampling, only one sample is taken and inferences about the population are made from the information in that sample alone. Thus, a sample of size n may be considered as one realization of many repeated samples of size n that generate a distribution of a sample statistic.

8.5 SAMPLING DISTRIBUTION OF THE MEAN

The concept of the sampling distribution of a mean is the same as the sampling distribution of a proportion. In Section 8.4 we found that we could describe the distribution of sample proportions (from repeated samples of the same size) both theoretically and empirically. We can also describe the distribution of sample means (from repeated samples of the same size) both theoretically and empirically.

Since the observation is a measure, each item in a large (or infinite) population has associated with it a value x. The distribution of these values in the population is called the **parent distribution** of x. This specifies the probability that, in a sample of size 1, x will lie between any two values c and d:

$$P(c < x < d).$$

Note that an interval is used rather than a given value since in a theoretically continuous distribution the probability that an observation x will be exactly equal to some value c is strictly 0:

$$P(x = c) = 0.$$

If a sample of n items is taken, we have n values of x (some of which may be the same). We can denote these sample values as x_1, $x_2, \ldots, x_n$. In condensing this information, we may choose to use the mean, $\bar{x}$ of the sample. Now the probability that $\bar{x}$ falls between two values c and d, i.e.,

$$P(c < \bar{x} < d),$$

Table 8.4. An empirical sampling distribution
of the mean in 100 repeated samples of size 10

$\bar{x}$	f
-∞ to -30.00	3
-29.99 to -10.00	30
-9.99 to 10.00	40
10.01 to 30.00	25
30.01 to ∞	2
Total	100

may be calculated from a knowledge of the parent distribution. These probabilities form the *theoretical sampling distribution* of the mean $\bar{x}$ (from repeated samples of size n). To get the empirical sampling distribution of the mean we take, say, 100 repeated but independent samples of size n. If $n = 10$, then each of these samples produces a value for $\bar{x}$ which we may tabulate as in Table 8.4.

In this section we have been concerned with the sampling distribution of the mean in repeated random samples of fixed size n. This follows from our choice of the mean as the statistic used to summarize the information in the sample. We may use other statistics such as the median, mode, range, standard deviation, or one of our own constructs to extract or to emphasize a certain characteristic of the data in a sample of size n. Again, there is no conceptual difference between the sampling distribution of the range in repeated random samples of size n and the sampling distribution of the mean. We may generate the sampling distribution for any summary statistic empirically by drawing repeated random samples and tabulating the resultant histogram of frequencies with which values of the chosen statistic are produced in a long series of samples of the same size. (Research statisticians rely heavily on this method to investigate the theoretical sampling distributions for statistics whose distributions are unknown.)

8.6 PROPERTIES OF SAMPLING DISTRIBUTIONS

A frequency distribution gives the frequency with which a value of a variable x occurs, either in a population or in a sample. A sampling distribution gives the frequency with which a value of a statistic, such as the sample mean, occurs either in an infinite or finite series of repeated samples of fixed size. The sampling distribution for a finite number of values for a sample statistic is an empirical sampling distribution and is similar to the frequency distribution of a variable x in a finite sample. The difference between a sampling distribution of a statistic and a frequency distribution of a variable *must* be kept clearly in mind if the reader is to understand the following developments, especially the concept of the standard error.

Although conceptually the sampling distribution is very different from the frequency distribution of a variable, we can apply the same procedures of summarizing a sampling distribution that we used in summarizing a frequency distribution. In particular, we can think of and calculate measures of central tendency and variation for sampling distributions just as we did for frequency distributions. Thus, we can talk about the mean, median, and mode of a given sample statistic and likewise the range or standard deviation of this statistic. Indeed we can conceive of the following combinations:

$$
\text{the}
\begin{cases}
\text{mean} \\
\text{median} \\
\text{mode} \\
\text{range} \\
\text{standard deviation}
\end{cases}
\text{of the}
\begin{cases}
\text{mean} \\
\text{median} \\
\text{mode} \\
\text{range} \\
\text{standard deviation}
\end{cases}
$$

in repeated random samples of constant size n. Thus we can discuss the mean range of the observations in repeated samples, and likewise the range of the means for the same set of samples.

Slightly changing our wording, we can call the standard deviation of a sample statistic the **standard error** of this statistic. This is a useful convention since, depending on the context, the mean is reported with either a standard deviation or a standard error. The *standard deviation* describes the variation of the measure about the mean, whereas the *standard error* of the mean describes the variation of sample means about the population mean. This distinction is often misunderstood or overlooked with the result that the variation in the original observations is grossly understated (as when the standard error is interpreted as a standard deviation) or that the sampling variation of the mean is grossly overstated (when the standard deviation is interpreted as a standard error).

Example.   The mean vital capacity in 80 repeated observations on one man was given as 4.5 ± 0.2 liters.

If 0.2 represents the standard deviation of the observations, then the standard error of the mean is approximately 0.02. (See Section 8.6.1 for this derivation.)

If, however, we erroneously conclude that 0.2 represents the standard error, we are too high by a factor of about 10 (in this case) and are grossly understating the precision of the mean 4.5 liters as an estimate of the man's "true" vital capacity.

8.6.1 Properties of the Sampling Distribution of the Mean

It is natural to summarize the sampling distribution of the mean by the mean of the sample means and by the standard error of the sample means. These measure, respectively, the location and dispersion of the sample means, which we now treat as our basic observations.

In the theoretical sampling distribution of the mean (as in the case where an infinite number of repeated random samples have been taken) the mean of these sample means is equal to the population mean:

$$\mathcal{E}(\bar{x}) = \mu.$$

This is what is meant by saying that the sample mean is an **unbiased estimator** of the population mean.

It may also be demonstrated that the standard error of a sample mean (which measures the variation of sample means about μ, the population mean) is related to the standard deviation (which measures the variation of the variable x about μ) by the equation

$$\sigma_{\bar{x}} = \sigma_x / \sqrt{n},$$

where

$\sigma_{\bar{x}}$ = the standard error of the mean,
$\sigma_{\bar{x}}$ = the standard deviation of x,
n = the constant sample size used in repeated sampling.

This is an extremely important result, since if we draw a random sample of nine observations from a population with a known standard deviation $\sigma_x = 0.15$, we can calculate the precision of this estimate of μ (i.e., how close $\bar{x}$ is to μ) by calculating the standard error of the mean from this relationship:

$$\sigma_{\bar{x}} = 0.15/\sqrt{9} = 0.05.$$

If this standard error is too large, we can decide to increase the size of the sample until we achieve the desired degree of accuracy.

Example. Given $\sigma_x = 0.15$, what sample size is required to give a standard error of the mean equal to 0.01?

Solve $0.01 = 0.15/\sqrt{n}$ to get $n = 225$.

Finally if the original variable x is normally distributed, the sampling distribution of $\bar{x}$ will also be normally distributed. Since we can calculate the mean and standard error for the sampling distribution from a knowledge of the population mean and standard deviation, the sampling distribution of the mean is completely specified. We summarize this in standard notation as follows:

$$\text{If } \quad x \sim N(\mu, \sigma), \quad \text{then} \quad \bar{x} \sim N(\mu, \sigma/\sqrt{n}),$$

where $\bar{x}$ is generated by repeated random samples of fixed size n. Even if x is not normally distributed, the sampling distribution of $\bar{x}$ will quickly tend toward a normal distribution as the fixed sample size increases.

We can use these properties to get confidence limits for μ based on a mean from a single sample. Assume that it is known that x is normally distributed with known standard deviation σ_x. Then if a random sample of size n is taken, it generates a sample mean $\bar{x}$ that is an estimate of μ. From the above properties, $\bar{x}$ will have values than are normally distributed around μ with standard error $\sigma_{\bar{x}} = \sigma_x/\sqrt{n}$.

Now, since the sampling distribution is normal, we know that $\mu \pm 1.96 \, \sigma_{\bar{x}}$ will contain 95% of all means (based on samples of size n). It may therefore be argued that in 95 samples out of 100 the values $\bar{x} \pm 1.96 \, \sigma_{\bar{x}}$ will contain μ. Therefore 95% confidence limits for the mean are given by

$$\bar{x} \pm 1.96 \; \sigma_x/\sqrt{n}$$

assuming that n, $\bar{x}$, and σ_x are known. When it is known only that the parent distribution is normally distributed, i.e., when σ_x is unknown, we can use the same argument and substitute s_x for σ_x. The standard deviation s_x is calculated from the sample. Because we are using an estimate of σ_x, we have less information than before, when σ_x was known, and our confidence limits will be wider. Therefore we use

$$\bar{x} \pm ts_{\bar{x}},$$

where $s_{\bar{x}}$ is an estimated standard error derived from $s_x/\sqrt{n}$ and t is a tabulated value which gets larger as the sample size n gets smaller. (As information decreases our confidence limits get wider.)

Even when the original or parent distribution is not normal, the above approach is often used. This use of a technique that assumes a normal distribution in situations where the parent distribution is non-normal relies on the approximation of the sampling distribution to the normal as the sample size increases. The use of this approach may be defended when the sample size is large, say $n > 50$. For $n \leqslant 50$ and for a non-normal distribution, a distribution-free technique may be used, such as that outlined in Section 8.2.

8.6.2 Properties of the Sampling Distribution of a Proportion

The underlying parent distribution for a proportion is the trivial one of $\mathcal{P}\%$ positives and $(1 - \mathcal{P})\%$ negatives. Therefore it is meaningless to talk about a population mean or a population standard deviation for the parent distribution. We simply have as the sole population parameter, where

$$\mathcal{P} = P(x = 1) = \text{probability of a positive}$$

and

$$1 - \mathcal{P} = P(x = 0) = \text{probability of a negative}.$$

However, for samples of size n, a sample proportion is the natural choice to summarize the information in a sample of a binomial variable. (This is all the information in the sample apart from the order in which the binomial values 0 and 1 occurred in the sample.)

Just as in the sampling distribution of a mean, the mean of repeated random sample proportions will equal the population proportion, i.e., $\mathcal{E}(p) = \mathcal{P}$. The standard error which measures the variation of sample proportions p about $\mathcal{P}$ in different samples of size n is conventionally derived as

$$\sigma_p = \sqrt{\frac{\mathcal{P}(1 - \mathcal{P})}{n}}$$

Also, for a fixed $\mathcal{P} = 0.5$ and as n increases, the sampling distribution tends toward the normal (p can take on more and more values as n increases and $1/n$ decreases).

Approximate 95% confidence limits for a proportion may be calculated as

$$p \pm 2\sqrt{\frac{p(1 - p)}{n}}.$$

The reader, however, is advised to use exact tables unless $np > 100$.

EXERCISES

8.1 A hospital corporation decides to build 5 hospitals, one in the 13 southern states, two in the 6 mid-Atlantic states, one in the 4 far western states, and one in either Michigan, Indiana, Illinois, or Wisconsin. Its officers have already selected a site in each state but want to choose the best combination of states in which to site the 5 hospitals subject to the above requirements. How many combinations of 5 sites have to be compared if no state may contain more than one new hospital?

8.2 The probability that a newborn baby will be a boy is 0.5. What family size is necessary to ensure with a probability of 95% that there will be at least one boy in the family?

8.3 Assume that boys and girls are equally likely in a family, and that the sex of the next child is independent of the sexes of earlier children. Representing a boy as B and a girl as G, list all types of 3-children families, and calculate the relative frequency of each type in the population of 3-children families. What is the probability that a family of size 3 will contain at least 2 girls?

8.4 A sample mean is given together with a value which is either the population standard deviation, the population standard error, the sample standard deviation, or the standard error estimated from the sample standard deviation. Explain how the various interpretations of this value alter its use in describing the sample mean.

8.5 A sample of 25 randomly chosen patients' bills will estimate the mean of all patients' bills with a standard error of $0.20. You would be satisfied with a standard error of $0.50. On the basis of this information, what is the minimum sample size which would give a standard error of $0.50?

FURTHER READING

Mainland, D. 1964. Elementary Medical Statistics. 2nd Ed. Chapter 11. W. B. Saunders Company, Philadelphia.

Maxwell, A. E. 1961. Analyzing Qualitative Data. Methuen, London. John Wiley & Sons, Inc., New York.

Noether, G. 1971. Introduction to Statistics: A Fresh Approach. Houghton Mifflin Company, Boston.

Sandler, H. E., and S. S. Stahl. 1959. Measurement of Periodontal Disease Prevalence. J. Amer. Dent. Ass. 58:93–97.

9
Significance Tests

9.1 WHAT IS A TEST OF SIGNIFICANCE?

The fact that this question has been delayed so long in this book, as in other textbooks, indicates how difficult it is to describe a test of significance in the absence of a background in statistical theory. It is hoped that the preceding chapters (especially Chapters 7 and 8) have now prepared the reader. However, since this chapter may be read without reference to those chapters, we shall first give an intuitive definition of a test of significance.

If 20 investigators carried out the same study independently of each other, and each used a 5% significance test to examine the validity of an assertion that was in fact true, only one (i.e., 1 in 20 or 5% on the average) would claim that the assertion was false. As an example, assume that each member of a 20-man jury used a 5% level of significance to "weigh the evidence." Note that the accused is assumed innocent until found guilty. Then only one juryman would vote "guilty" when *in fact* that accused was innocent (Feinberg, 1971).

A significance test may also be considered in terms of repeated identical studies done by the same investigator. If he repeated his study (whether it be an experiment or a survey) 20 times, each time starting *completely* from the beginning and using a 5% level of significance to judge his results, then, on an average, in one study out of the 20 he would conclude that his original premise was false, when it was in fact true. Now we consider an investigator who is going to do only *one* study. Before he begins, we can tell him that, if he uses a 5% significance test to evaluate his data, he will have a probability of 5% of erroneously concluding that the assumption on which he based the test was false when in fact it is true.

You can see how we are approaching the concept of a confidence limit. Indeed the 5% significance test is analogous to the 95% confidence limit. The difference is that in the calculation of confidence limits we work from the sample statistic to imputed values of a population parameter, whereas in a test of significance we start from an *assumed* value of the population parameter and calculate what would have been the likelihood of finding the observed value for the sample statistic. If this likelihood or probability is low, e.g., below 5%, we reject our assumed parameter value since we cannot discard the observed value of the sample statistic.

Example.   I tell you that I have a friend who is a normal adult male. What population does he belong to? A natural answer would be that he is American (since the author of the question is American). Now we test this assumption by measuring his height to test the assertion. Note that we are assuming that my friend is a random sample of 1 from the population of normal adult males in the United States. His height is 5 foot 2 inches. Given that the heights of normal adult males in America have a known distribution, we can calculate the probability of drawing a sample of one height which is as small or smaller than 5 foot 2 inches, and we find that this is 2%, i.e., $P = 2\%$. We then either have to accept that the sample is atypical in that men as small or smaller than 5 foot 2 inches only constitute 2% of the population (of normal adult American males), or (and this is the procedure followed) agree that, if the probability of getting a sample as small or smaller than 5 foot 2 inches is less than 5%, we reject our assumption that the man comes from the population of normal adult American males.

In statistical jargon, our test is significant at the 5% level. In this particular example the test worked correctly since my friend is a member of a North African tribe of pygmies. However, the test could have falsely rejected a true assumption since there are some normal adult American males who are 5 foot 2 inches or less in height.

The question arises, how do we know what assumption to make before proceeding with the test of significance? This depends on the context. In the above example, if the investigator had been working among pygmies the null hypothesis would have been different. The null hypothesis is defined in terms of what is the usual or standard experience in that situation. For example, although 98.6°F is known to be the usual body temperature, the mean temperature of a sample of fever patients would be expected to be higher. In other words, the population from which the sample is drawn will provide the parameters to be used in the null hypothesis. In addition, it is conventional to use the status quo until it has been shown (by a test of significance or otherwise) to be inappropriate. Thus, the assertion has been made by a former Secretary of Health that comprehensive health plans greatly reduce medical costs. To test this assertion we would sample a number of comprehensive health plans, get a combined average for the total cost of coverage, and compare this with current national figures generated by conventional methods of providing health care. The null hypothesis would be that comprehensive health plans provide health care at the same costs as traditional methods. This assumption would be rejected only if the sample mean from comprehensive plans were so much lower than standard costs as to be unlikely to have arisen by sampling variation. Note that if the costs of comprehensive care were found to be significantly less than standard health care costs we would then seek to rule out selection and other biases before accepting the Secretary's statement.

9.2   THE MEANING OF $P < 0.05$

It is fashionable to use statistical tests of significance even when they are unnecessary. Significance tests and confidence limits are appropriate only when a sample of independent observations has been *randomly* selected from a well-defined population. For the most part, this is not done. Therefore, it is advocated by Mainland

and others that the phrase "if the sample were randomly selected" be added to the interpretation of tests of significance and confidence limits. Otherwise, tests of significance can be made to appear to support anything by suitable manipulation of the data. Thus, at one time we could "prove" that adult males in London, England, were taller than adult males in the rest of that country by measuring the heights of a random sample of policemen. In London one had to be tall to join the police force and, therefore, policemen were atypical of the adult male population.

Also, it is inappropriate to use tests of significance to compare populations. Thus it would be inappropriate to apply a test of significance to test the truth of the statement, "patients in East Coast hospitals are significantly older than patients in West Coast hospitals." The addition of the recommended phrase "if the samples were randomly selected" demonstrates this, for clearly the samples were the very opposite of randomly selected. Rather, this is an example of the partition of a population (all United States hospitals) into subpopulations. The comparison of subpopulations is made directly. "Patients in East Coast hospitals are, on the average, three months older than patients in West Coast hospitals."

The use of 5% as the level of significance is entirely conventional, as is the use of 95% confidence limits. Just as the confidence levels of a set of confidence limits can be increased from 95% to 99%, so also can we adjust the level of significance from, say, 5% to 1%. In the latter case, we are imposing a more stringent criterion that may in fact render the procedure useless. Just as increasing the confidence level to 99% may result in confidence limits so wide that they are uninformative, so may a 1% level of significance result in our misclassifying real differences as being due to sampling variation; i.e., we shall miss those smaller real differences that would have been detected by a 5% test.

Conversely, a 70% confidence limit may be encouragingly narrow but at a risk that the parameter will fall outside these limits 3 times out of 10. In addition, a 30% test of significance (i.e., $P < 0.30$) will turn up an encouragingly larger number of "significant" results but a large fraction of these will be "false alarms" due to sampling variation. The level to be used in confidence limits, or in a test of significance, is therefore determined by the investigator before the analysis, and should reflect his standards and the use to which he plans to put the results. Thus, in a screening test of charges levied by different medical insurers, we might agree to use a 20% significance level, since companies that appear to have significantly higher charges will be further investigated and many of the cases of "significantly" higher charging will be found to be isolated examples untypical of that company. On the other hand, in attempting to decide whether or not to stop payment on those charges that appear to be "significantly" higher than the norm, a medical insurer may use a $P < 0.01$ level of significance, because of the embarassment and loss of good will that might result from an unsuccessful law suit.

Significance tests occur infrequently in management situations but they tend to be used often by investigators in experiments and surveys. The administrator rarely experiments with the system he controls (see Chapter 10). He may wish to test an idea or a hypothesis from time to time by drawing a sample or making a survey. A P value may therefore be calculated for what appears to be the appropriate significance test, but a test of significance is strictly appropriate only when the information used is a *random* sample from a well-defined population. (One exception here is the χ^2 test of independence in a contingency table. See Section 9.7.2.) In the majority of applications, the data will not be randomly selected. All we can say, therefore, if told that a *nonrandom* sample mean of patient charges for a given hospital is significantly higher ($P < 0.05$) than the national average, is that this finding is unlikely to be due to chance alone. However, the sample of charges may well be unrepresentative of the hospital, which in terms of all its charges (the population) may be, in fact, below the national norms as given in the Hospitals Administration Services (HAS) program of the American Hospitals Association.

9.3 CATALOG OF TESTS OF SIGNIFICANCE

One of the most difficult aspects of data analysis is the selection of the correct procedure from among the various tests available.

For this reason, it is useful to categorize tests of significance according to:

   the type of variable (a measure or classification),
   the number of samples to be compared (one, two, or more
      than two),
   the total number of observations, and
   whether auxiliary parameters are known or estimated.

This information and the hypothesis specified may be used to determine the **test statistic** to be calculated from the sample or samples. The probability of finding a value as deviant as or more deviant than the test statistic, on the basis of the underlying assumption, is derived from the appropriate table. This table gives the probabilities associated with different test statistics. These tables in fact are based on the sampling distribution of the test statistic. If the probability associated with the test statistic is less than the level of significance, then the test is said to be significant and the null hypothesis is rejected in favor of the alternative hypothesis. All of this assumes, of course, that the sample(s) is (are) randomly selected from a well-defined population.

In the following sections we describe a few of the more common and useful tests of significance. We begin by considering tests of means from one or two samples. Testing the means from more than two samples requires an analysis of variance that is outside the scope of this book. In Sections 9.4 and 9.5, tests of significance are given for testing a mean or means in a variety of situations.

9.4   TESTS OF THE MEAN FROM
A SINGLE SAMPLE (NORMAL DISTRIBUTION)

9.4.1   Sample Size Not More than 20; Standard Deviation in the Population Unknown

Assume that we want to test whether the population mean μ is a specified value, say 27. We draw a random sample of size n where n is less than or equal to 20, e.g., $n = 18$. Further, although we know that the basic observation x is a continuous measure that

Table 9.1. Significance limits for the (absolute) difference of a sample mean $\bar{x}$ from its population mean μ in a random sample of size n drawn from a normally distributed population

$$\text{Test statistic} = \frac{|\bar{x} - \mu|}{x_{(n)} - x_{(1)}} \, .$$

n	P					
	0.10	0.05	0.02	0.01	0.002	0.001
2	3.157	6.353	15.910	31.828	159.16	318.31
3	0.885	1.304	2.111	3.008	6.77	9.58
4	0.529	0.717	1.023	1.316	2.29	2.85
5	0.388	0.507	0.685	0.843	1.32	1.58
6	0.312	0.399	0.523	0.628	0.92	1.07
7	0.263	0.333	0.429	0.507	0.71	0.82
8	0.230	0.288	0.366	0.429	0.59	0.67
9	0.205	0.255	0.322	0.374	0.50	0.57
10	0.186	0.230	0.288	0.333	0.44	0.50
11	0.170	0.210	0.262	0.302	0.40	0.44
12	0.158	0.194	0.241	0.277	0.36	0.40
13	0.147	0.181	0.224	0.256	0.33	0.37
14	0.138	0.170	0.209	0.239	0.31	0.34
15	0.131	0.160	0.197	0.224	0.29	0.32
16	0.124	0.151	0.186	0.212	0.27	0.30
17	0.118	0.144	0.177	0.201	0.26	0.28
18	0.113	0.137	0.168	0.191	0.24	0.26
19	0.108	0.131	0.161	0.182	0.23	0.25
20	0.104	0.126	0.154	0.175	0.22	0.24

From *Documenta Geigy Scientific Tables*, 7th ed., 1971, p. 53, by permission of the publishers Ciba-Geigy Ltd., Basel, Switzerland.

follows a normal distribution (approximately), we do not know the value of σ, the standard deviation in the parent distribution.

In this situation we may use Table 9.1, which gives probabilities for the test statistic

$$\frac{|\bar{x} - \mu|}{x_{(n)} - x_{(1)}} \, .$$

This test statistic is derived by dividing the absolute difference between the sample mean $\bar{x}$ and the hypothetical population mean μ by the sample range, calculated as the difference between the largest sample value $x_{(n)}$ and the smallest sample value $x_{(1)}$. This statistic, calculated for the sample, yields a value that is then compared with the value of the statistic (derived from the table) for the specified significance level and sample size.

Example. We wish to test whether the pH level (acidity versus alkalinity) of plaques (tooth deposits) in persons who have no caries (tooth decay) is either acid or alkali. (The pH of distilled water is 7.0.) We take a random sample of 18 persons who have no carious teeth and measure the pH level of plaques taken from their teeth. We find that our 18 observations or values of x have a mean of 7.4 pH units and a range of 2.4 pH units, from 6.2 to 8.6.

Let us first establish the tabulated value of the test statistic. For a 5% significance level and a sample size of 18, Table 9.1 gives a value of 0.137. (Make sure that you agree before reading on.) Now, if the test statistic is greater than 0.137, we shall say that the test is significant and conclude that the pH level of plaque in caries-free persons is significantly different from our hypothesized values of 7.0. Conversely, if the sample test statistic is less than 0.137, we shall conclude that the test is nonsignificant at the 5% level and retain our assumption that the pH level of plaque in caries-free persons is 7.0 (neutral).

We are now prepared not only to calculate the test statistic but also to interpret the result. Since we may assign to μ the value 7.0, and since we know that $x_{(n)} - x_{(1)} = 2.4$, we have

$$\frac{|\bar{x} - \mu|}{x_{(n)} - x_{(1)}} = \frac{7.4 - 7.0}{2.4} = \frac{0.4}{2.4} = 0.167.$$

Since this value is greater than the tabulated value of 0.137, we conclude that the test is significant and, since the sample mean is 7.4, that there is some evidence that plaque pH levels are higher than 7.0 in caries-free persons.

An alternative use of Table 9.1 is to calculate the test statistic as 0.167 and to enter the table at $n = 18$ to get the probability associated with this value of the test statistic. The table gives

a test statistic value of 0.168 associated with $P = 0.02$,
a test statistic value of 0.137 associated with $P = 0.05$.

Our test statistic of 0.167 falls between these, so we may attach a probability of between 5% and 2% to the test statistic and write

$$0.05 > P > 0.02 \quad \text{or} \quad 0.02 < P < 0.05.$$

Since we are using a 5% level of significance and since the P value associated with the test statistic is less than this, the test is significant. In this context this means that the probability of finding a mean of 7.4 or higher (or its converse, a mean of 6.6 or lower) in a random sample of 18 observations from a normally distributed population in which the true mean is 7.0 is between 5% and 2%. Since this probability is less than our criterion of 5%, we conclude not that this sample is a freak, but that our assumption of μ = 7.0 is wrong. Similarly, if the probability associated with the test statistic as read from the table is greater than 5%, then the opposite argument applies, i.e., the test is nonsignificant, the sample could well have arisen by chance from a population with μ = 7.0, and, therefore, we retain μ = 7.0.

9.4.2 Sample Size Not More than 100; Population Standard Deviation σ Unknown

Table 9.1 covers samples up to 20 observations. What if the sample size is greater than 20? In this case we use a test statistic called t. The table of probabilities for values of t is given in Table 9.2.

This test statistic is defined as

$$t = \frac{|\bar{x} - \mu|}{s/\sqrt{n}},$$

where, as before, $\bar{x}$ is the sample mean, μ is the hypothetical population mean, and $|\bar{x} - \mu|$ is the absolute difference between them. The denominator is formed by dividing s, the sample standard deviation, by $\sqrt{n}$, the square root of the sample size.

Note that for the t statistic, we must calculate the standard deviation s for the sample as well as the mean $\bar{x}$. Apart from using a different test statistic and table, the test of significance is calculated as in Section 9.4.1. We shall use Table 9.2 in several different situations (see § 9.5.2, Unequal Sample Sizes or Samples Greater than 20; Standard Deviations Unknown but Assumed Equal). In order to facilitate multiple usage of the table, Table 9.2 is given in terms of the number of **degrees of freedom** ν where ν

Statistical Principles in Health Care Information

Table 9.2. Significance levels for the (absolute) difference of a sample mean $\bar{x}$ from its population mean μ in a random sample of size n from a normally distributed population

$$\text{Test statistic} = t = \frac{|\bar{x} - \mu|}{s/\sqrt{n}}$$

Significance level

ν	0.20	0.10	0.05	0.025	0.02	0.01	0.005	0.001
1	3.078	6.3138	12.706	25.452	31.821	63.657	127.32	636.619
2	1.886	2.9200	4.3027	6.2053	6.965	9.9248	14.089	31.598
3	1.638	2.3534	3.1825	4.1765	4.541	5.8409	7.4533	12.924
4	1.533	2.1318	2.7764	3.4954	3.747	4.6041	5.5976	8.610
5	1.476	2.0150	2.5706	3.1634	3.365	4.0321	4.7733	6.869
6	1.440	1.9432	2.4469	2.9687	3.143	3.7074	4.3168	5.959
7	1.415	1.8946	2.3646	2.8412	2.998	3.4995	4.0293	5.408
8	1.397	1.8595	2.3060	2.7515	2.896	3.3554	3.8325	5.041
9	1.383	1.8331	2.2622	2.6850	2.821	3.2498	3.6897	4.781
10	1.372	1.8125	2.2281	2.6338	2.764	3.1693	3.5814	4.587
11	1.363	1.7959	2.2010	2.5931	2.718	3.1058	3.4966	4.437
12	1.356	1.7823	2.1788	2.5600	2.681	3.0545	3.4284	4.318
13	1.350	1.7709	2.1604	2.5326	2.650	3.0123	3.3725	4.221
14	1.345	1.7613	2.1448	2.5096	2.624	2.9768	3.3257	4.140
15	1.341	1.7530	2.1315	2.4899	2.602	2.9467	3.2860	4.073
16	1.337	1.7459	2.1199	2.4729	2.583	2.9208	3.2520	4.015
17	1.333	1.7396	2.1098	2.4581	2.567	2.8982	3.2225	3.965
18	1.330	1.7341	2.1009	2.4450	2.552	2.8784	3.1966	3.922
19	1.328	1.7291	2.0930	2.4334	2.539	2.8609	3.1737	3.883
20	1.325	1.7247	2.0860	2.4231	2.528	2.8453	3.1534	3.850
21	1.323	1.7207	2.0796	2.4138	2.518	2.8314	3.1352	3.819
22	1.321	1.7171	2.0739	2.4055	2.508	2.8188	3.1188	3.792
23	1.319	1.7139	2.0687	2.3979	2.500	2.8073	3.1040	3.767
24	1.318	1.7109	2.0639	2.3910	2.492	2.7969	3.0905	3.745
25	1.316	1.7081	2.0595	2.3846	2.485	2.7874	3.0782	3.725
26	1.315	1.7056	2.0555	2.3788	2.479	2.7787	3.0669	3.707
27	1.314	1.7033	2.0518	2.3734	2.473	2.7707	3.0565	3.690
28	1.313	1.7011	2.0484	2.3685	2.467	2.7633	3.0469	3.674
29	1.311	1.6991	2.0452	2.3638	2.462	2.7564	3.0380	3.659
30	1.310	1.6973	2.0423	2.3596	2.457	2.7500	3.0298	3.646
31	1.3095	1.6955	2.0395	2.3556	2.453	2.7441	3.0222	3.6338
32	1.3086	1.6939	2.0370	2.3519	2.449	2.7385	3.0150	3.6221
33	1.3078	1.6924	2.0345	2.3484	2.445	2.7333	3.0083	3.6111
34	1.3070	1.6909	2.0323	2.3451	2.441	2.7284	3.0020	3.6011
35	1.3062	1.6896	2.0301	2.3420	2.438	2.7239	2.9962	3.5915
36	1.3055	1.6883	2.0281	2.3391	2.434	2.7195	2.9905	3.5824
37	1.3049	1.6871	2.0262	2.3364	2.431	2.7155	2.9853	3.5741
38	1.3042	1.6860	2.0244	2.3338	2.428	2.7116	2.9804	3.5661
39	1.3037	1.6849	2.0227	2.3313	2.426	2.7079	2.9757	3.5586
40	1.3031	1.6839	2.0211	2.3290	2.423	2.7045	2.9713	3.5511
41	1.3026	1.6829	2.0196	2.3268	2.421	2.7012	2.9671	3.5446
42	1.3020	1.6820	2.0181	2.3247	2.418	2.6981	2.9631	3.5383
43	1.3016	1.6811	2.0167	2.3226	2.416	2.6952	2.9592	3.5323
44	1.3011	1.6802	2.0154	2.3207	2.414	2.6923	2.9556	3.5264
45	1.3007	1.6794	2.0141	2.3189	2.412	2.6896	2.9522	3.5207
46	1.3002	1.6787	2.0129	2.3172	2.410	2.6870	2.9489	3.5153
47	1.2998	1.6779	2.0118	2.3155	2.408	2.6846	2.9457	3.5104
48	1.2994	1.6772	2.0106	2.3139	2.406	2.6822	2.9427	3.5053
49	1.2991	1.6766	2.0096	2.3124	2.405	2.6800	2.9398	3.5010
50	1.2987	1.6759	2.0086	2.3109	2.403	2.6778	2.9370	3.4965

(Cont'd)

Table 9.2 (*Continued*)

ν	Significance level							
	0.20	0.10	0.05	0.025	0.02	0.01	0.005	0.001
51	1.2984	1.6753	2.0077	2.3096	2.402	2.6758	2.9344	3.4924
52	1.2981	1.6747	2.0067	2.3082	2.400	2.6738	2.9318	3.4883
53	1.2978	1.6742	2.0058	2.3070	2.399	2.6719	2.9295	3.4845
54	1.2975	1.6736	2.0049	2.3057	2.397	2.6700	2.9271	3.4807
55	1.2972	1.6731	2.0041	2.3045	2.396	2.6683	2.9249	3.4770
56	1.2969	1.6725	2.0033	2.3033	2.395	2.6666	2.9226	3.4733
57	1.2967	1.6721	2.0025	2.3022	2.393	2.6650	2.9205	3.4702
58	1.2964	1.6716	2.0017	2.3011	2.392	2.6633	2.9184	3.4670
59	1.2962	1.6712	2.0010	2.3001	2.391	2.6618	2.9165	3.4638
60	1.2959	1.6707	2.0003	2.2991	2.390	2.6603	2.9146	3.4606
61	1.2957	1.6703	1.9997	2.2982	2.389	2.6590	2.9128	3.4577
62	1.2954	1.6698	1.9990	2.2972	2.388	2.6576	2.9110	3.4548
63	1.2952	1.6694	1.9984	2.2963	2.387	2.6563	2.9094	3.4521
64	1.2950	1.6690	1.9977	2.2954	2.386	2.6549	2.9077	3.4494
65	1.2948	1.6687	1.9972	2.2946	2.385	2.6537	2.9061	3.4470
66	1.2945	1.6683	1.9966	2.2937	2.384	2.6525	2.9045	3.4445
67	1.2944	1.6680	1.9961	2.2929	2.383	2.6513	2.9031	3.4423
68	1.2942	1.6676	1.9955	2.2921	2.382	2.6501	2.9016	3.4400
69	1.2940	1.6673	1.9950	2.2914	2.381	2.6491	2.9002	3.4378
70	1.2938	1.6669	1.9945	2.2907	2.381	2.6480	2.8988	3.4355
71	1.2936	1.6666	1.9940	2.2900	2.380	2.6470	2.8976	3.4333
72	1.2934	1.6663	1.9935	2.2893	2.379	2.6459	2.8963	3.4310
73	1.2933	1.6660	1.9931	2.2887	2.378	2.6450	2.8950	3.4291
74	1.2931	1.6657	1.9926	2.2880	2.378	2.6440	2.8937	3.4272
75	1.2930	1.6655	1.9922	2.2874	2.377	2.6431	2.8925	3.4253
76	1.2928	1.6652	1.9917	2.2867	2.376	2.6421	2.8913	3.4234
77	1.2927	1.6649	1.9913	2.2861	2.376	2.6413	2.8903	3.4217
78	1.2925	1.6646	1.9909	2.2855	2.375	2.6404	2.8892	3.4200
79	1.2924	1.6644	1.9905	2.2850	2.374	2.6396	2.8882	3.4185
80	1.2922	1.6641	1.9901	2.2844	2.374	2.6388	2.8871	3.4169
81	1.2921	1.6639	1.9897	2.2839	2.373	2.6380	2.8861	3.4152
82	1.2920	1.6637	1.9893	2.2833	2.372	2.6372	2.8851	3.4135
83	1.2919	1.6635	1.9890	2.2828	2.372	2.6365	2.8842	3.4121
84	1.2917	1.6632	1.9886	2.2823	2.371	2.6357	2.8832	3.4106
85	1.2916	1.6630	1.9883	2.2818	2.371	2.6350	2.8823	3.4091
86	1.2915	1.6628	1.9880	2.2813	2.370	2.6343	2.8814	3.4076
87	1.2914	1.6626	1.9877	2.2809	2.370	2.6336	2.8805	3.4063
88	1.2913	1.6624	1.9873	2.2804	2.369	2.6329	2.8796	3.4050
89	1.2912	1.6622	1.9870	2.2800	2.369	2.6323	2.8788	3.4036
90	1.2910	1.6620	1.9867	2.2795	2.368	2.6316	2.8779	3.4022
91	1.2909	1.6618	1.9864	2.2791	2.368	2.6310	2.8772	3.4010
92	1.2908	1.6616	1.9861	2.2787	2.367	2.6303	2.8764	3.3997
93	1.2907	1.6614	1.9859	2.2783	2.367	2.6298	2.8757	3.3986
94	1.2906	1.6612	1.9856	2.2779	2.366	2.6292	2.8749	3.3975
95	1.2905	1.6611	1.9853	2.2775	2.366	2.6286	2.8742	3.3964
96	1.2904	1.6609	1.9850	2.2771	2.366	2.6280	2.8734	3.3952
97	1.2904	1.6608	1.9848	2.2768	2.365	2.6275	2.8728	3.3940
98	1.2903	1.6606	1.9845	2.2764	2.365	2.6270	2.8721	3.3928
99	1.2902	1.6604	1.9843	2.2761	2.364	2.6265	2.8714	3.3919
100	1.2901	1.6602	1.9840	2.2757	2.364	2.6260	2.8707	3.3909

From *Documenta Geigy Scientific Tables,* 7th ed., 1971, pp. 32-33, by permission of the publishers Ciba-Geigy Ltd., Basel, Switzerland.

will be defined differently in each situation using Table 9.2. In this application,

$$\nu = n - 1$$

This reduction of the sample size by one recognizes the fact that to calculate s, the sample standard deviation, we first have to calculate $\bar{x}$, the sample mean. There are therefore only $(n - 1)$ independent deviations from $\bar{x}$ in a sample of size n.

Example. Blood specimens are taken from 55 elderly persons. This sample of 55 is considered to be representative of the population of elderly persons living independently in a given public health district. These blood samples are assayed spectrographically for iron content (to measure the extent of anemia) at the Public Health Center. In a healthy person the iron content in plasma is about 0.19 mg/100 ml, so we assume that $\mu = 0.19$.

The value of t given by Table 9.2, $\nu = 54$ and $P = 0.05$, is 2.0049 and we shall now calculate the value of the t test statistic in the sample. The sample of 55 estimations (one for each person) has a mean of 0.17 and a standard deviation of 0.06. The value of the t statistic in the sample is, therefore,

$$t = \frac{|\, 0.17 - 0.19 \,|}{0.06/\sqrt{55}}$$

$$= \frac{0.02}{0.008}$$

$$= 2.50.$$

This sample value of t is larger than 2.0049 and the test is, therefore, significant, the mean iron content of 55 blood specimens being significantly less than normal. This suggests that old people living alone in this district have lower iron concentrations in their blood than others. Whether this is called anemia is, of course, a matter of definition.

Alternatively, we can enter Table 9.2 with the value of the test statistic ($t = 2.50$). Reading along the row headed $\nu = 54$, we find that this value of t has a probability between 0.02 and 0.01. Therefore the probability of finding a random sample of size 55, yielding a mean as far from the normal μ of 0.19 as this value of 0.17, is

$$0.02 > P > 0.01 \quad \text{or} \quad 0.01 < P < 0.02.$$

Since this probability is less than 0.05, we consider the assumption of $\mu = 0.19$ to be untenable; i.e., the information in the sample tends to invalidate the assumption that this population mean is 0.19 mg/100 ml. Therefore, either the population is anemic or our standard is wrong.

Note. A person familiar with statistical inference would say that the above test is incorrectly described as a **double-tailed** t test rather than as a **single-tailed** t test. What does this jargon mean in terms of the above example? This 5% significance test is a double-tailed test since both high and low sample means are considered significant in rejecting the original hypothesis

$$\mu = 0.19.$$

In a single-tailed test of significance, however, the original hypothesis is of the form

$$\mu \leqslant \mu_0$$

and we reject this only if the sample mean exceeds the critical value or, alternately,

$$\mu_0 \leqslant \mu$$

and we reject this only if the sample mean is lower than the critical value.

In the above example we are only interested in anemia, i.e., a lowering of the iron concentration in the blood. Therefore, the original hypothesis (which we set out of test) should be

$$\mu \geqslant 0.19 \quad \text{rather than} \quad \mu = 0.19.$$

If, for example, the mean of the 55 blood specimens had been 0.215, we would not have done the test since a sample mean of 0.215 is consistent with a population mean of 0.19 or higher. Our 5% significance test, therefore, is composed of a 2.5% significance test against a higher than normal mean and a 2.5% significance test against a lower than normal mean. If we are interested only in detecting whether old people living alone have adequate or inadequate levels of iron in their blood, then we can use $\mu = 0.19$ as before, but use a tabulated t value of 1.6736. For $\nu = 54$ this is the value of t associated with a double-tailed test at a 10% level of significance composed of two single-tailed tests at the 5% level of significance. In our example, the calculated value of t from the sample was 2.50. Comparing this with 1.6736, the 5% level of a single t test still gives us a significant test. Indeed, we now estimate P to lie between 0.01 and 0.005. Thus by eliminating one alternative, $\bar{x} > \mu$, we have made the test more sensitive in the detection of anemia.

9.4.3   Population Standard Deviation Known or Sample Size Greater

Consider a measureable variable x that follows a normal distribution for which μ is specified by the hypothesis and σ is known. In this case we use as the test statistic z, where z is defined as

$$z = \frac{|\bar{x} - \mu|}{\sigma/\sqrt{n}}.$$

This is just the t statistic with the known value of the population standard deviation σ in place of s, the sample standard deviation. As before, z is evaluated by substituting sample values (here only $\bar{x}$ and n) into the test statistic. The table used is Table 9.3, which gives the probability associated with values of z as large as or larger than the specified value. Note, however, that Table 9.3 is unlike the previous two tables in that P, the probability associated with z, does not vary with sample size so there is no column for n or degrees of freedom in the table.

Example.   The daily costs of operating a hospital are known for the past year. These 365 observations appear to follow a normal distribution with $\mu = \$30,000$ and $\sigma = \$3,600$. At the end of the current year, the hospital administrator selects 13 days at random. He is prepared to assume that these 13 days will be a representative sample of the 365 days of the current year and that the daily costs of the current year will follow a normal distribution with standard deviation $\sigma = \$3,600$, the same as last year's. He wants to determine whether there is any evidence to suggest whether his

Table 9.3. Probability that the (absolute) value of z is as great as or greater than the value given, where $z = |\bar{x} - \mu|/(\sigma/\sqrt{n})$

$P \rightarrow$ $\downarrow$	0.00	0.01	0.02	0.03	0.04	0.05	0.06	0.07	0.08	0.09
0.0	∞	2.575829	2.326348	2.170090	2.053749	1.959964	1.880794	1.811911	1.750686	1.695398
0.1	1.644854	1.598193	1.554774	1.514102	1.475791	1.439531	1.405072	1.372204	1.340755	1.310579
0.2	1.281552	1.253565	1.226528	1.200359	1.174987	1.150349	1.126391	1.103063	1.080319	1.058122
0.3	1.036433	1.015222	0.994458	0.974114	0.954165	0.934589	0.915365	0.896473	0.877896	0.859617
0.4	0.841621	0.823894	0.806421	0.789192	0.772193	0.755415	0.738847	0.722479	0.706303	0.690309
0.5	0.674490	0.658838	0.643345	0.628006	0.612813	0.597760	0.582842	0.568051	0.553385	0.538836
0.6	0.524401	0.510073	0.495850	0.481727	0.467699	0.453762	0.439913	0.426148	0.412463	0.398855
0.7	0.385320	0.371856	0.358459	0.345126	0.331853	0.318639	0.305481	0.292375	0.279319	0.266311
0.8	0.253347	0.240426	0.227545	0.214702	0.201893	0.189118	0.176374	0.163658	0.150969	0.138304
0.9	0.125661	0.113039	0.100434	0.087845	0.075270	0.062707	0.050154	0.037608	0.025069	0.012533

From *Documenta Geigy Scientific Tables,* 7th ed., 1971, p. 31, by permission of the publishers Ciba-Geigy Ltd., Basel, Switzerland.

average daily costs are higher or lower than last year's average costs.

Table 9.3 gives a $z = 1.96$ equivalent to a $P = 0.05$ (in a double-tailed test of significance). The mean of 13 days' cost is $31,500. Evaluating z we get

$$z = \frac{|\bar{x} - \mu|}{\sigma/\sqrt{n}}$$

$$= \frac{|\,\$31,500 - \$30,000\,|}{\$3,600/\sqrt{13}}$$

$$= 1.50,$$

which is less than 1.96. The test, therefore, is not significant (i.e., there is insufficient evidence with this size of sample to discard the assumption that average daily costs have changed over the past year).

Note. If the test had been significant, the conclusion would have been that chance or sampling fluctuations constituted an unlikely explanation for the significantly high or low sample mean of 13 daily costs. This may have meant that average daily costs had changed, but there are alternative explanations:

1) that our assumption that $\sigma = \$3,600$ was wrong,
2) that the 13 days were nonrepresentative of the current year with regard to daily cost of running the hospital, or
3) that the 365 daily costs do not follow a normal distribution.

Note that the above procedure can be followed when σ is unknown if the sample size is large ($n > 100$). The reason for this is that, in a large sample, s is a very close estimate of σ. In other words, we can find out what σ is by calculating the standard deviation in a large random sample. Note also that t and z are similarly defined except that t uses s whereas z contains σ. As s becomes a better estimate of σ (as the sample size increases), the test statistic t approaches the test statistic z. This fact is reflected in the tables. The 5% level of z is 1.96 and examination of Table 9.2 confirms that the 5% level of t approaches this as n and therefore ν increases. Indeed, for a sample of size 100, the t value corresponding to $P = 0.05$ is already 1.98, and for a sample of size 200, $t = 1.97$, so there is little approximation in using Table 9.3 instead of Table 9.2 extended for samples > 100.

9.5 TEST OF THE DIFFERENCE
BETWEEN TWO SAMPLE MEANS (NORMAL DISTRIBUTION)

9.5.1 Sample Sizes Equal and Not More than 20; Standard Deviations Unknown but Assumed Equal

If we are interested in a measurable variable x that is normally distributed, and if we have drawn two random samples of the same size ($n \leqslant 20$), we may wish to test whether these samples come from a common population with common mean μ or from two populations with different means μ', μ'', where $\mu' \neq \mu''$.

The test statistic here is

$$\frac{|\bar{x}' - \bar{x}''|}{x'_{(n)} - x'_{(1)} + x''_{(n)} - x''_{(1)}}$$

where $|\bar{x}' - \bar{x}''|$ is the absolute difference between the two sample means and where this is divided by the sum of the two sample ranges.

Note here that we arbitrarily designate the observations in one sample as

$$x'_{(1)}, x'_{(2)}, x'_{(3)}, \ldots, x'_{(n)}$$

in increasing order of their size and the ordered observations in the second sample as

$$x''_{(1)}, x''_{(2)}, x''_{(3)}, \ldots, x''_{(n)}$$

with means $\bar{x}'$ and $\bar{x}''$, respectively. The denominator of the test statistic,

$$x'_{(n)} - x'_{(1)} + x''_{(n)} - x''_{(1)},$$

is therefore the largest value in the first sample minus the smallest value in the first sample plus the largest value in the second sample minus the smallest value in the second sample. Table 9.4 gives the probabilities associated with this test statistic for given sizes of samples up to 20.

Implicit in the numerator of this test statistic and others that follow in this section is a zero term. This zero term represents the difference between μ' and μ''. Thus, the numerator is really

$$(\bar{x}' - \mu') - (\bar{x}'' - \mu'') = (\bar{x}' - \bar{x}'') - (\mu' - \mu'')$$

Table 9.4. Significance limits for the (absolute) difference between two sample means derived from independent random samples of the same size n drawn from a normally distributed population

$$\text{Test statistic} = \frac{|\bar{x}' - \bar{x}''|}{x_{(n)}' - x_{(1)}' + x_{(n)}'' - x_{(1)}''}$$

	Significance level					
n	0.10	0.05	0.02	0.01	0.002	0.001
2	1.161	1.714	2.777	3.958	8.91	12.62
3	0.487	0.636	0.857	1.047	1.64	2.09
4	0.322	0.407	0.524	0.619	0.87	1.00
5	0.247	0.307	0.386	0.448	0.61	0.68
6	0.203	0.250	0.311	0.357	0.47	0.52
7	0.174	0.213	0.263	0.300	0.39	0.43
8	0.153	0.187	0.230	0.261	0.34	0.37
9	0.137	0.167	0.205	0.232	0.30	0.32
10	0.125	0.152	0.186	0.210	0.27	0.29
11	0.117	0.140	0.170	0.192	0.24	0.26
12	0.107	0.130	0.158	0.178	0.22	0.24
13	0.101	0.122	0.147	0.166	0.21	0.22
14	0.095	0.114	0.138	0.156	0.20	0.21
15	0.090	0.108	0.131	0.147	0.18	0.20
16	0.085	0.103	0.124	0.139	0.17	0.19
17	0.081	0.098	0.118	0.132	0.17	0.18
18	0.078	0.094	0.113	0.126	0.16	0.17
19	0.075	0.090	0.108	0.121	0.15	0.16
20	0.072	0.086	0.104	0.116	0.15	0.16

From *Documenta Geigy Scientific Tables,* 7th ed., 1971, p. 53, by permission of the publishers Ciba-Geigy Ltd., Basel, Switzerland.

but since $\mu' = \mu''$ by assumption, the latter term is zero. Whereas in a single sample we had to specify the value of μ in our hypothesis, in testing differences between two means it is sufficient simply to specify their difference, i.e., zero.

The procedures of the test follow the same pattern as in a single sample test. A level of significance is first chosen. This and the common sample size determine a **critical value** for the test statistic derived from the table. The test statistic is then calculated from the sample and compared with the critical value. If the test statistic is greater than the critical value, the test is called significant and the conclusion is reached that there is a significant difference between the two population means μ' and μ''. Conversely, if the test statistic is smaller than the critical value, the test is considered to be nonsignificant and the assumption that both samples come from the same population is retained.

Example. Shafer, Hine, and Levy (1963) compared the pH levels of stimulated saliva in caries-free and high-caries children from 8½ to 9 years of age. The sample statistics (slightly modified) were as follows:

Sample	Number	Mean	Range
Caries-free	12	7.44	7.13–7.77
High-caries	12	7.41	7.02–7.71

Table 9.4 gives, for $n = 12$ and $P = 0.05$, a critical value of the test statistic of 0.130. Evaluating the test statistic, we get

$$\frac{|x' - x''|}{x'_{(n)} - x'_{(1)} + x''_{(n)} - x''_{(1)}} = \frac{|7.44 - 7.41|}{7.77 - 7.13 + 7.71 - 7.02}$$

$$= \frac{0.03}{0.64 + 0.69}$$

$$= 0.0225,$$

which is less than the critical value of 0.130. Therefore, there is no ground (contrary to the impression given by the authors) to reject our basic assumption that the mean pH level of stimulated saliva was the same in 8-year-old children with and without caries (if a 5% level of significance is acceptable).

9.5.2 Unequal Sample Sizes or Samples Greater than 20; Standard Deviations Unknown but Assumed Equal

Again we assume that the samples are drawn randomly either from a common population with a normal distribution or from two populations whose normal distributions differ only in the mean. The test statistic used in this situation is a two-sample variant of the single-sample t test statistic and is also called t. (No ambiguity arises since it should be obvious from the context whether we mean the one-sample or the two-sample case.)

The two-sample t test statistic is defined as

$$t = \frac{\mid \bar{x}' - \bar{x}'' \mid}{\sqrt{\frac{(s')^2}{n'} + \frac{(s'')^2}{n''}}}.$$

This expression has the same numerator as above, namely the absolute value of the difference of the two sample means. The denominator is the square root of the sum of the squared sample standard deviations divided by the sample sizes, where s' and s'' are the sample standard deviations in the first and second samples, respectively.

We may use Table 9.2 by entering the table with degrees of freedom calculated as

$$\nu = n' + n'' - 2.$$

Example. The suggestion has been made that two physicians working in a comprehensive health plan have different methods of prescribing drugs for their patients. Since it was realized that different patients need varying amounts of drugs, it was decided to randomize the referral of a certain class of patients to the two doctors in the next week and to measure the costs of drugs prescribed for each patient. The physicians agreed to this but were unaware of the criterion used except that, as ever, each patient was to be given that treatment necessary for his recovery and maintenance of health.

At the end of the period, 63 patients who met "the criteria" had been allocated to the two physicians, one seeing 28 patients and the other 35. The results of the trial were as follows:

$$n' = 28, \quad \bar{x}' = \$13.16, \quad s' = \$4.04,$$

$$n'' = 35, \quad \bar{x}'' = \$15.10, \quad s'' = \$3.57.$$

To test whether this trial is indicative of a real difference in prescribing habits rather than a chance phenomenon, we use the t test statistic for two samples. First, we look up the critical value of t for a 5% level of significance in Table 9.2. To do this we enter the table with degrees of freedom

$$\begin{aligned} \nu &= n' + n'' - 2 = 28 + 35 - 2 \\ &= 63 - 2 \\ &= 61 \end{aligned}$$

and find that

$$t = 1.9997.$$

We now calculate the t statistic as

$$\begin{aligned} t &= \frac{|\bar{x}' - \bar{x}''|}{\sqrt{\dfrac{(s')^2}{n'} + \dfrac{(s'')^2}{n''}}} \\[2mm] &= \frac{|13.16 - 15.10|}{\sqrt{\dfrac{(4.04)^2}{28} + \dfrac{(3.57)^2}{35}}} \\[2mm] &= \frac{1.94}{\sqrt{0.9471}} \\[2mm] &= \frac{1.94}{0.97} \\[2mm] &= 2.00. \end{aligned}$$

Now this value of t appears to be just slightly greater than the tabulated value corresponding to a 5% probability. Therefore, we might say that the test is significant and that there does appear to be a real difference in the prescribing habits of the two physicians.

However, the value of t calculated from the data was expressed only to two decimal places. If we calculated it to four decimal points to conform to the number of places given in the table, then we might reach a different conclusion. All we can really say is that the probability of a difference as large as or larger than that observed between the two doctors' average levels of drug costs occurring by chance is about 5%. The test of significance, therefore, is inconclusive. This situation is comparable to that of a hung jury. Just as a retrial is ordered in the case of a hung jury, so another test is required here.

It is not, however, advocated that one or more additional observations be taken and added to the original samples for recalculation. This is equivalent to making a decision on these additional data, just as adding an additional juryman to a hung jury would result in *his* deciding the guilt or innocence of the accused, at least in those situations where a majority vote was required.

Note. In this situation, the test is slightly improved if the common standard deviation is estimated by pooling both samples as follows:

$$s^2 = \frac{(n' - 1)(s')^2 + (n'' - 1)(s'')^2}{n' + n'' - 2}$$

The denominator for t then becomes

$$\sqrt{\frac{s^2}{n'} + \frac{s^2}{n''}}$$

For the situation in which it cannot be assumed that $(s')^2$ and $(s'')^2$ estimate the same variance, see Snedecor and Cochran's *Statistical Methods,* 6th Edition, Section 4.14.

Example.

$$n' = 28 \quad s' = 4.04$$
$$n'' = 35 \quad s'' = 3.57$$
$$s^2 = \frac{(28-1) \times (4.04)^2 + (35-1) \times (3.57)^2}{28 + 35 - 2}$$

$$= \frac{27 \times 16.3216 + 34 \times 12.7449}{61}$$

$$= \frac{440.6832 + 433.3266}{61}$$

$$= \frac{874.0098}{61}$$

$$= 14.3280$$

$$\sqrt{\frac{s^2}{n'} + \frac{s^2}{n''}} = \sqrt{\frac{14.3280}{28} + \frac{14.3280}{35}}$$

$$= \sqrt{0.5117 + 0.4094}$$

$$= \sqrt{0.9211}$$

$$= 0.96$$

$$t = \frac{1.94}{0.96} = 2.02$$

The test statistic has increased very slightly by pooling. Since the critical value is 1.9997 or 2.00 to two decimal places we have shown that the difference is just significant at the 5% level by pooling the two sample standard deviations.

9.5.3 Population Standard Deviations σ' and σ'' Known, or Sample Sizes n' and n'' Both Greater than 100 (Normal Distribution)

In the one sample case, we can substitute σ for s in the test statistic when σ is known or estimated without error and then use tables for z. In the two-sample case also, we can substitute estimates for the true values of the standard deviations. The two-sample version of z is

$$z = \frac{|\bar{x}' - \bar{x}''|}{\sqrt{\frac{(\sigma')^2}{n'} + \frac{(\sigma'')^2}{n''}}}$$

and this is evaluated using Table 9.3.

Example. A random sample of 120 Veterans Administration hospitals was selected, along with a random sample of 150 university hospitals. For each of these hospitals the number of vacancies for nurses on July 1 was noted. We treat the number of vacancies as a continuous variable following a normal distribution and test whether there is a significant difference (at the 5% level) in the mean number of vacancies in the two types of hospitals.

We know from Table 9.3 that the critical value of z corresponding to $P = 0.05$ is 1.96. The statistics from the two samples are

V.A. hospitals: $n' = 120$, $\bar{x}' = 21.3$, $s' = 4.8$,

university hospitals: $n'' = 150$, $\bar{x}'' = 26.6$, $s'' = 4.5$.

We evaluate z by substituting s' for σ' and s'' for σ'' since these are estimated from samples greater than 100:

$$z = \frac{|\, 21.3 - 26.6\,|}{\sqrt{\dfrac{(4.8)^2}{120} + \dfrac{(4.5)^2}{150}}} = \frac{5.6}{\sqrt{0.3270}} = \frac{5.6}{0.57} \approx 10.$$

If our assumptions are correct, there is little doubt that, in the total population of hospitals, university hospitals had a higher mean number of vacancies for nurses than V.A. hospitals on July 1.

9.6   TESTS OF UNDERLYING ASSUMPTIONS

In single samples we assume that the observations are independent of each other, i.e., the size of one observation does not affect the size of another and that the variable follows a normal distribution. In tests on two samples we assume, in addition, that the two population standard deviations σ' and σ'' are identical in value. We may check these assumptions by using the tests below.

9.6.1   Test of Outliers

Perhaps the most common departure from the normal distribution is the occurrence of extreme values caused by errors in observation or by gross errors in recording, transmitting, or copying data. To detect whether or not an observation is an outlier, we can apply a test of significance based on the normal distribution. In a small sample ($n \leqslant 25$) for which the population mean μ and standard

Table 9.5. Significance limits for testing extreme values of a sample from a normally distributed population (Values of x arranged so that $x_{(1)} \leqslant x_{(2)} \leqslant x_{(3)} \leqslant \cdots \leqslant x_{(n)}$.)

| | P (Single Tail) | | | | | | | |
n	0.30	0.20	0.10	0.05	0.02	0.01	0.005	Test statistic
3	0.684	0.781	0.886	0.941	0.976	0.988	0.994	
4	471	560	679	765	846	889	926	$x_{(n)} - x_{(n-1)}$
5	373	451	557	642	729	780	821	————————
6	318	386	482	560	644	698	740	$x_{(n)} - x_{(1)}$
7	281	344	434	507	586	637	680	
8	0.318	0.385	0.479	0.554	0.631	0.683	0.725	$x_{(n)} - x_{(n-1)}$
9	288	352	441	512	587	635	677	————————
10	265	325	409	477	551	597	639	$x_{(n)} - x_{(2)}$
11	0.391	0.442	0.517	0.576	0.638	0.679	0.713	$x_{(n)} - x_{(n-2)}$
12	370	419	490	546	605	642	675	————————
13	351	399	467	521	578	615	649	$x_{(n)} - x_{(2)}$
14	0.370	0.421	0.492	0.546	0.602	0.641	0.674	
15	353	402	472	525	579	616	647	
16	338	386	454	507	559	595	624	
17	325	373	438	490	542	577	605	
18	314	361	424	475	527	561	589	
19	304	350	412	462	514	547	575	$x_{(n)} - x_{(n-2)}$
20	0.295	0.340	0.401	0.450	0.502	0.535	0.562	————————
21	287	331	391	440	491	524	551	$x_{(n)} - x_{(3)}$
22	280	323	382	430	481	514	541	
23	274	316	374	421	472	505	532	
24	268	310	367	413	464	497	524	
25	262	304	360	406	457	489	516	

From *Documenta Geigy Scientific Tables*, 7th ed., 1971, p. 53, by permission of the publishers Ciba-Geigy Ltd., Basel, Switzerland.

deviation σ are unknown, we may use Table 9.5, which gives single-tailed probability values associated with an outlier on the large size. (To test whether a very small value is an outlier, we simply rank the observations from largest to smallest instead of from smallest to largest.) The test is conducted like other tests of significance, by assuming, to start with, that the suspected value is a member of the population from which the sample is drawn.

Example. A random sample of 18 hospitals is selected, and their staffing ratio (number of professionals per 100 inpatients) is recorded as follows (in decreasing order): 28, 25, 22, 21, 21, 20, 20, 19, 19, 19, 18, 18, 17, 15, 15, 13, 12, 6. To test whether 6 is an outlier at the 5% level of significance (single-tailed), we consult Table 9.5 and find that the test statistic is, for a sample of size 18,

$$\frac{x_{(n)} - x_{(n-2)}}{x_{(n)} - x_{(3)}}$$

and that this takes a value of 0.475 for $P = 0.05$. Evaluating the test statistic in the sample we get

$$\frac{x_{(n)} - x_{(n-2)}}{x_{(n)} - x_{(3)}} = \frac{6 - 13}{6 - 22} = 0.4375,$$

which is smaller than the critical value of 0.475. Therefore, the test is nonsignificant, and we conclude that a value as low as 6 professionals per 100 inpatients is a possible value from a population that follows a normal distribution and that produced the observed sample. (Note that the test of 28 as an outlier would have yielded a sample test statistic of

$$\frac{28 - 22}{28 - 13} = 0.4000,$$

which again is not significant at the 5% level.)

If the parameters μ and σ are known for the normal distribution from which the sample is derived, we can use

$$\frac{|x_{(n)} - \mu|}{\sigma}$$

as test statistic and use Table 9.3 to get the (double-tailed) probability of observations as deviant as $x_{(n)}$ from the mean. Thus, if

$$\frac{|x_{(n)} - \mu|}{\sigma} > 1.96$$

then the probability of observations as extreme or more extreme than $x_{(n)}$ (in either direction) will be less than 5%.

When μ and σ are unknown we may use an approximate test for samples greater than 25 by substituting sample estimates of the mean and standard deviation for μ and σ in the text sketched above. The approximation involved in using

$$\frac{|x_{(n)} - \bar{x}|}{s}$$

rather than

$$\frac{|x_{(n)} - \mu|}{\sigma}$$

in conjunction with Table 9.3 will improve as the sample size increases.

Note that if Table 9.3 is used to test for outliers in one direction only, then a 5% single-tailed test will be achieved by using a critical value of 1.64, since this is equivalent to a double-tailed test with 10% significance.

Other types of departures from normality exist and may be verified by other specific or general tests. Also, departures from other assumed frequency distributions may be detected by either specific or general tests of "goodness to fit." (See Section 9.7.2 for a description of the χ^2 test, which may be used to test "goodness of fit.")

9.6.2 Test for Dependence between Successive Observations

One of the most frequently broken assumptions in statistical analysis is that observations generated sequentially in time can be treated as though they are independent. In general, independence is a function of the underlying mechanism producing the observations and of the time interval between observations.

The coefficient of **serial correlation** measures the degree of association between observations. We illustrate the procedure by a test of independence between successive observations.

The test statistic is the sum of squares of differences between successive observations x_i, x_{i+1} divided by the sum of squares of deviations of the observations from the mean. This may be written as

$$\frac{\sum_{i=1}^{n-1} (x_{i+1} - x_i)^2}{\sum_{i=1}^{n} (x_i - \bar{x})^2}.$$

Note that in this notation we number the observations as they occur $x_1, x_2, \ldots, x_n$. Critical values of this statistic are tabulated in Table 9.6. In effect, two single-tailed tests of significance are tabulated, since upper and lower critical values of the test statistic are given. If the test statistic exceeds the larger of the two critical

Table 9.6. Significance limits P for a test of the randomness of successive observations in a sample of size n drawn from a normally distributed population.

$$\text{Test statistic} = \sum_{1}^{n-1} (x_{i+1} - x_i)^2 \bigg/ \sum_{1}^{n} (x_i - \bar{x})^2$$

n	$P = 0.10$	$P = 0.02$	n	$P = 0.10$	$P = 0.02$
			101	1.676-2.324	1.542-2.458
			102	677- 323	544- 456
			103	679- 321	546- 454
4	0.780-3.220	0.626-3.374	104	680- 320	548- 452
5	0.820-3.180	0.538-3.462	105	1.682-2.318	1.550-2.450
6	890- 110	561- 439	106	683- 317	552- 448
7	936- 064	614- 386	107	685- 315	554- 446
8	982- 018	663- 337	108	686- 314	556- 444
9	1.024-2.976	709- 291	109	688- 312	558- 442
10	1.062-2.938	0.752-3.248	110	1.689-2.311	1.560-2.440
11	096- 904	791- 209	111	691- 309	562- 438
12	128- 872	828- 172	112	692- 308	564- 436
13	156- 844	862- 138	113	693- 307	566- 434
14	182- 818	893- 107	114	695- 305	568- 432
15	1.205-2.795	0.922-3.078	115	1.696-2.304	1.570-2.430
16	227- 773	949- 051	116	697- 303	572- 428
17	247- 753	974- 026	117	698- 302	573- 427
18	266- 734	998- 002	118	700- 300	575- 425
19	283- 717	1.020-2.980	119	701- 299	577- 423
20	1.300-2.700	1.041-2.959	120	1.702-2.298	1.579-2.421
21	315- 685	060- 940	121	703- 297	580- 420
22	329- 671	078- 922	122	705- 295	582- 418
23	342- 658	096- 904	123	706- 294	584- 416
24	355- 645	112- 888	124	707- 293	585- 415
25	1.367-2.633	1.128-2.872	125	1.708-2.292	1.587-2.413
26	378- 622	142- 858	126	709- 291	589- 411
27	389- 611	157- 843	127	710- 290	590- 410
28	399- 601	170- 830	128	711- 289	592- 408
29	409- 591	183- 817	129	713- 287	593- 407
30	1.418-2.582	1.195-2.805	130	1.714-2.286	1.595-2.405
31	426- 574	207- 793	131	715- 285	597- 403
32	435- 565	218- 782	132	716- 284	598- 402
33	443- 557	228- 772	133	717- 283	600- 400
34	451- 549	239- 761	134	718- 282	601- 399
35	1.458-2.542	1.248-2.752	135	1.719-2.281	1.602-2.398
36	466- 534	258- 742	136	720- 280	604- 396
37	472- 528	267- 733	137	721- 279	605- 395
38	479- 521	276- 724	138	722- 278	607- 393
39	486- 514	285- 715	139	723- 277	608- 392
40	1.492-2.508	1.293-2.707	140	1.724-2.276	1.610-2.390
41	498- 502	302- 698	141	725- 275	611- 389
42	504- 496	310- 690	142	726- 274	612- 388
43	510- 490	317- 683	143	727- 273	614- 386
44	515- 485	325- 675	144	728- 272	615- 385
45	1.521-2.479	1.332-2.668	145	1.729-2.271	1.616-2.384
46	526- 474	339- 661	146	730- 270	618- 382
47	530- 470	345- 655	147	730- 270	619- 381
48	535- 465	351- 649	148	731- 269	620- 380
49	539- 461	357- 643	149	732- 268	621- 379
50	1.544-2.456	1.363-2.637	150	1.733-2.267	1.623-2.377
51	548- 452	368- 632	151	734- 266	624- 376
52	552- 448	374- 626	152	735- 265	625- 375
53	556- 444	379- 621	153	736- 264	626- 374
54	559- 441	384- 616	154	737- 263	627- 373
55	1.563-2.437	1.390-2.610	155	1.737-2.263	1.629-2.371
56	567- 433	395- 605	156	738- 262	630- 370
57	571- 429	400- 600	157	739- 261	631- 369
58	574- 426	405- 595	158	740- 260	632- 368
59	578- 422	410- 590	159	741- 259	633- 367
60	1.581-2.419	1.414-2.586	160	1.742-2.258	1.634-2.366
61	584- 416	419- 581	161	742- 258	636- 364
62	587- 413	423- 577	162	743- 257	637- 363
63	590- 410	427- 573	163	744- 256	638- 362
64	593- 407	431- 569	164	745- 255	639- 361
65	1.596-2.404	1.435-2.565	165	1.745-2.255	1.640-2.360
66	599- 401	439- 561	166	746- 254	641- 359
67	602- 398	443- 557	167	747- 253	642- 358
68	605- 395	447- 553	168	748- 252	643- 357
69	608- 392	451- 549	169	748- 252	644- 356
70	1.611-2.389	1.454-2.546	170	1.749-2.251	1.645-2.355
71	614- 386	458- 542	171	750- 250	646- 354
72	617- 383	461- 539	172	751- 249	647- 353
73	620- 380	465- 535	173	751- 249	648- 352
74	623- 377	468- 532	174	752- 248	649- 351
75	1.625-2.375	1.471-2.529	175	1.753-2.247	1.650-2.350
76	628- 372	474- 526	176	753- 247	651- 349
77	630- 370	477- 523	177	754- 246	652- 348
78	632- 368	480- 520	178	755- 245	653- 347
79	635- 365	483- 517	179	755- 245	654- 346
80	1.637-2.363	1.486-2.514	180	1.756-2.244	1.655-2.345
81	639- 361	489- 511	181	757- 243	656- 344
82	641- 359	492- 508	182	757- 243	657- 343
83	643- 357	495- 505	183	758- 242	658- 342
84	645- 355	498- 502	184	759- 241	659- 341
85	1.647-2.353	1.501-2.499	185	1.759-2.241	1.660-2.340
86	649- 351	504- 496	186	760- 240	661- 339
87	651- 349	507- 493	187	761- 239	662- 338
88	653- 347	510- 490	188	761- 239	662- 338
89	655- 345	512- 488	189	762- 238	663- 337
90	1.657-2.343	1.515-2.485	190	1.763-2.237	1.664-2.336
91	659- 341	518- 482	191	763- 237	665- 335
92	661- 339	520- 480	192	764- 236	666- 334
93	662- 338	523- 477	193	764- 236	667- 333
94	664- 336	525- 475	194	765- 235	668- 332
95	1.666-2.334	1.528-2.472	195	1.766-2.234	1.668-2.332
96	668- 332	530- 470	196	766- 234	669- 331
97	669- 331	532- 468	197	767- 233	670- 330
98	671- 329	535- 465	198	767- 233	671- 329
99	673- 327	537- 463	199	768- 232	672- 328
100	1.674-2.326	1.539-2.461	200	1.768-2.232	1.673-2.327
			∞	2.000-2.000	2.000-2.000

From *Documenta Geigy Scientific Tables*, 7th ed., 1971, p. 58, by permission of the publishers Ciba-Geigy Ltd., Basel, Switzerland.

values in the $P = 0.10$ column, then we conclude that the test is significant and that there is evidence at the 5% level of significance that the observations are being influenced by some short-term cyclic influences. If, on the other hand, the test statistic falls below the smaller of the two critical values, we conclude that the test is significant at the 5% level and that there is evidence of a trend in the data over time. (Additional tests for randomness in serial observations are given in Section 11.7.)

Example. A week was chosen at random from the previous year and the number of occupied beds in a given hospital recorded for each of the seven days. The observations were 98, 103, 105, 105, 102, 101, 100 for the seven days, Sunday through Saturday. To test whether we may consider these as a sample of independent observations, we calculate

$$\frac{\sum_{i=1}^{6} (x_{i+1} - x_i)^2}{\sum_{i=1}^{7} (x_i - \bar{x})^2}$$

$$= \frac{[(98-103)^2 + (103-105)^2 + (105-105)^2 + (105-102)^2 + (102-101)^2 + (101-100)^2]}{[(98-\bar{x})^2) + (103-\bar{x})^2 + (105-\bar{x})^2 + (105-\bar{x})^2 + (102-\bar{x})^2 + (101-\bar{x})^2 + (100-\bar{x})^2]}.$$

Now $\bar{x} = 102$, so that the test statistic evaluated from the sample has a value of $40/40 = 1.000$, which falls between the tabulated values of 0.936 and 3.064. Therefore, in spite of an apparent cycle over the week, the test has failed to demonstrate this as a real characteristic of the population of weeks. We conclude that there is insufficient evidence to reject our original assumption of independence of the observations. This, of course, may be a case of insufficient information to demonstrate a week-long cycle. Two or three weeks' data would presumably give a significant test, if each week demonstrated the same midweek peak.

9.6.3 Test of Equality of Two Standard Deviations

Two random samples provide us with independent estimates of what we assume to be a common standard deviation (at least in tests of the two sample means). To test this assumption, that both s' and s'' estimate a common σ, we use the F test (so named after Sir Ronald, formerly R. A., Fisher, the English statistician).

The test statistic is simply the ratio of the squares of the two sample standard deviations. Conventionally we divide the larger by the smaller and perform a test of significance. Table 9.7 gives the 5% critical value ($P = 0.05$) for the F statistic according to the sizes of the two samples (n', n''). Thus

$$F = \frac{(s')^2}{(s'')^2}$$

where s' is the larger standard deviation, and n' is the size of the sample in which this is calculated, s'' is the smaller standard deviation, and n'' is the size of the sample in which this is calculated.

If the F statistic calculated from the two samples is greater than the critical value of F, then the test is significant at the 5% level and the assumption that both s' and s'' estimate a common standard deviation is rejected. The examples below explain when to use a single-tailed test (Table 9.7a) and when to use a double-tailed test (Table 9.7b).

Example. An illness is characterized by wildly fluctuating temperatures. Each hour the temperatures of two hospitalized patients, one of whom is suspected of having the illness, are recorded; it is known that the other patient does not have the illness.

The sample size is 11 for the patient with the more variable temperature (one observation was indecipherable on the chart) and 12 for the control patient without this disease. The two standard deviations based on 11 and 12 observations, respectively, were 1.4°F and 0.7°F, so that

$$F = \frac{(1.4)^2}{(0.7)^2} = 4$$

and

$$n' = 11, \qquad n'' = 12.$$

Since we are interested in determining whether the suspected patient's temperature is more variable than the control patient's, we use a single tail test. Table 9.7a gives a critical value of $F = 2.85$ corresponding to a one-tailed 5% level of significance and 11 and 12 observations, respectively. The implied assumption in this test

Table 9.7 Five percent significance for F, the ratio of the larger sample variance to the smaller, based on random samples of size n' and n'' respectively from a normally distributed population.

a) Single tail

n'' \ n'	2	3	4	5	6	7	8	9	10	11	13	16	21	25	31	41	61	121	∞
2	161.4	199.5	215.7	224.6	230.2	234.0	238.9	240.5	241.9	243.9	245.9	248.0	249.1	250.1	251.1	252.2	253.3	254.3	
3	18.51	19.00	19.16	19.25	19.30	19.33	19.35	19.37	19.38	19.40	19.41	19.43	19.45	19.45	19.46	19.47	19.48	19.49	19.50
4	10.13	9.55	9.28	9.12	9.01	8.94	8.89	8.85	8.81	8.79	8.74	8.70	8.66	8.64	8.62	8.59	8.57	8.55	8.53
5	7.71	6.94	6.59	6.39	6.26	6.16	6.09	6.04	6.00	5.96	5.91	5.86	5.80	5.77	5.75	5.72	5.69	5.66	5.63
6	6.61	5.79	5.41	5.19	5.05	4.95	4.88	4.82	4.77	4.74	4.68	4.62	4.56	4.53	4.50	4.46	4.43	4.40	4.36
7	5.99	5.14	4.76	4.53	4.39	4.28	4.21	4.15	4.10	4.06	4.00	3.94	3.87	3.84	3.81	3.77	3.74	3.70	3.67
8	5.59	4.74	4.35	4.12	3.97	3.87	3.79	3.73	3.68	3.64	3.57	3.51	3.44	3.41	3.38	3.34	3.30	3.27	3.23
9	5.32	4.46	4.07	3.84	3.69	3.58	3.50	3.44	3.39	3.35	3.28	3.22	3.15	3.12	3.08	3.04	3.01	2.97	2.93
10	5.12	4.26	3.86	3.63	3.48	3.37	3.29	3.23	3.18	3.14	3.07	3.01	2.94	2.90	2.86	2.83	2.79	2.75	2.71
11	4.96	4.10	3.71	3.48	3.33	3.22	3.14	3.07	3.02	2.98	2.91	2.85	2.77	2.74	2.70	2.66	2.62	2.58	2.54
12	4.84	3.98	3.59	3.36	3.20	3.09	3.01	2.95	2.90	2.85	2.79	2.72	2.65	2.61	2.57	2.53	2.49	2.45	2.40
13	4.75	3.89	3.49	3.26	3.11	3.00	2.91	2.85	2.80	2.75	2.69	2.62	2.54	2.51	2.47	2.43	2.38	2.34	2.30
14	4.67	3.81	3.41	3.18	3.03	2.92	2.83	2.77	2.71	2.67	2.60	2.53	2.46	2.42	2.38	2.34	2.30	2.25	2.21
15	4.60	3.74	3.34	3.11	2.96	2.85	2.76	2.70	2.65	2.60	2.53	2.46	2.39	2.35	2.31	2.27	2.22	2.18	2.13
16	4.54	3.68	3.29	3.06	2.90	2.79	2.71	2.64	2.59	2.54	2.48	2.40	2.33	2.29	2.25	2.20	2.16	2.11	2.07
17	4.49	3.63	3.24	3.01	2.85	2.74	2.66	2.59	2.54	2.49	2.42	2.35	2.28	2.24	2.19	2.15	2.11	2.06	2.01
18	4.45	3.59	3.20	2.96	2.81	2.70	2.61	2.55	2.49	2.45	2.38	2.31	2.23	2.19	2.15	2.10	2.06	2.01	1.96
19	4.41	3.55	3.16	2.93	2.77	2.66	2.58	2.51	2.46	2.41	2.34	2.27	2.19	2.15	2.11	2.06	2.02	1.97	1.92
20	4.38	3.52	3.13	2.90	2.74	2.63	2.54	2.48	2.42	2.38	2.31	2.23	2.16	2.11	2.07	2.03	1.98	1.93	1.88
21	4.35	3.49	3.10	2.87	2.71	2.60	2.51	2.45	2.39	2.35	2.28	2.20	2.12	2.08	2.04	1.99	1.95	1.90	1.84
22	4.32	3.47	3.07	2.84	2.68	2.57	2.49	2.42	2.37	2.32	2.25	2.18	2.10	2.05	2.01	1.96	1.92	1.87	1.81
23	4.30	3.44	3.05	2.82	2.66	2.55	2.46	2.40	2.34	2.30	2.23	2.15	2.07	2.03	1.98	1.94	1.89	1.84	1.78
24	4.28	3.42	3.03	2.80	2.64	2.53	2.44	2.37	2.32	2.27	2.20	2.13	2.05	2.01	1.96	1.91	1.86	1.81	1.76
25	4.26	3.40	3.01	2.78	2.62	2.51	2.42	2.36	2.30	2.25	2.18	2.11	2.03	1.98	1.94	1.89	1.84	1.79	1.73
26	4.24	3.39	2.99	2.76	2.60	2.49	2.40	2.34	2.28	2.24	2.16	2.09	2.01	1.96	1.92	1.87	1.82	1.77	1.71
27	4.23	3.37	2.98	2.74	2.59	2.47	2.39	2.32	2.27	2.22	2.15	2.07	1.99	1.95	1.90	1.85	1.80	1.75	1.69
28	4.21	3.35	2.96	2.73	2.57	2.46	2.37	2.31	2.25	2.20	2.13	2.06	1.97	1.93	1.88	1.84	1.79	1.73	1.67
29	4.20	3.34	2.95	2.71	2.56	2.45	2.36	2.29	2.24	2.19	2.12	2.04	1.96	1.91	1.87	1.82	1.77	1.71	1.65
30	4.18	3.33	2.93	2.70	2.55	2.43	2.35	2.28	2.22	2.18	2.10	2.03	1.94	1.90	1.85	1.81	1.75	1.70	1.64
31	4.17	3.32	2.92	2.69	2.53	2.42	2.33	2.27	2.21	2.16	2.09	2.01	1.93	1.89	1.84	1.79	1.74	1.68	1.62
41	4.08	3.23	2.84	2.61	2.45	2.34	2.25	2.18	2.12	2.08	2.00	1.92	1.84	1.79	1.74	1.69	1.64	1.58	1.51
61	4.00	3.15	2.76	2.53	2.37	2.25	2.17	2.10	2.04	1.99	1.92	1.84	1.75	1.70	1.65	1.59	1.53	1.47	1.39
121	3.92	3.07	2.68	2.45	2.29	2.17	2.09	2.02	1.96	1.91	1.83	1.75	1.66	1.61	1.55	1.50	1.43	1.35	1.25
∞	3.84	3.00	2.60	2.37	2.21	2.10	2.01	1.94	1.88	1.83	1.75	1.67	1.57	1.52	1.46	1.39	1.32	1.22	1.00

160

b) Double tail

n''＼n'	2	3	4	5	6	7	8	9	10	11	13	16	21	25	31	41	61	121	∞
2	647.8	799.5	864.2	899.6	921.8	937.1	948.2	956.7	963.3	968.6	976.7	984.9	993.1	997.2	1001	1006	1010	1014	1018
3	38.51	39.00	39.17	39.25	39.30	39.33	39.36	39.37	39.39	39.40	39.41	39.43	39.45	39.46	39.46	39.47	39.48	39.49	39.50
4	17.44	16.04	15.44	15.10	14.88	14.73	14.62	14.54	14.47	14.42	14.34	14.25	14.17	14.12	14.08	14.04	13.99	13.95	13.90
5	12.22	10.65	9.98	9.60	9.36	9.20	9.07	8.98	8.90	8.84	8.75	8.66	8.56	8.51	8.46	8.41	8.36	8.31	8.26
6	10.01	8.43	7.76	7.39	7.15	6.98	6.85	6.76	6.68	6.62	6.52	6.43	6.33	6.28	6.23	6.18	6.12	6.07	6.02
7	8.81	7.26	6.60	6.23	5.99	5.82	5.70	5.60	5.52	5.46	5.37	5.27	5.17	5.12	5.07	5.01	4.96	4.90	4.85
8	8.07	6.54	5.89	5.52	5.29	5.12	4.99	4.90	4.82	4.76	4.67	4.57	4.47	4.42	4.36	4.31	4.25	4.20	4.14
9	7.57	6.06	5.42	5.05	4.82	4.65	4.53	4.43	4.36	4.30	4.20	4.10	4.00	3.95	3.89	3.84	3.78	3.73	3.67
10	7.21	5.71	5.08	4.72	4.48	4.32	4.20	4.10	4.03	3.96	3.87	3.77	3.67	3.61	3.56	3.51	3.45	3.39	3.33
11	6.94	5.46	4.83	4.47	4.24	4.07	3.95	3.85	3.78	3.72	3.62	3.52	3.42	3.37	3.31	3.26	3.20	3.14	3.08
12	6.72	5.28	4.63	4.28	4.04	3.88	3.76	3.66	3.59	3.53	3.43	3.33	3.23	3.17	3.12	3.06	3.00	2.94	2.88
13	6.55	5.10	4.47	4.12	3.89	3.73	3.61	3.51	3.44	3.37	3.28	3.18	3.07	3.02	2.96	2.91	2.85	2.79	2.72
14	6.41	4.97	4.35	4.00	3.77	3.60	3.48	3.39	3.31	3.25	3.15	3.05	2.95	2.89	2.84	2.78	2.72	2.66	2.60
15	6.30	4.86	4.24	3.89	3.66	3.50	3.38	3.29	3.21	3.15	3.05	2.95	2.84	2.79	2.73	2.67	2.61	2.55	2.49
16	6.20	4.77	4.15	3.80	3.58	3.41	3.29	3.20	3.12	3.06	2.96	2.86	2.76	2.70	2.64	2.59	2.52	2.46	2.40
17	6.12	4.69	4.08	3.73	3.50	3.34	3.22	3.12	3.05	2.99	2.89	2.79	2.68	2.63	2.57	2.51	2.45	2.38	2.32
18	6.04	4.62	4.01	3.66	3.44	3.28	3.16	3.05	2.98	2.92	2.82	2.72	2.62	2.56	2.50	2.44	2.38	2.32	2.25
19	5.98	4.56	3.95	3.61	3.38	3.22	3.10	3.01	2.93	2.87	2.77	2.67	2.56	2.50	2.44	2.38	2.32	2.26	2.19
20	5.92	4.51	3.90	3.56	3.33	3.17	3.05	2.96	2.88	2.82	2.72	2.62	2.51	2.45	2.39	2.33	2.27	2.20	2.13
21	5.87	4.46	3.86	3.51	3.29	3.13	3.01	2.91	2.84	2.77	2.68	2.57	2.46	2.41	2.35	2.29	2.22	2.16	2.09
22	5.83	4.42	3.82	3.48	3.25	3.09	2.97	2.87	2.80	2.73	2.64	2.53	2.42	2.37	2.31	2.25	2.18	2.11	2.04
23	5.79	4.38	3.78	3.44	3.22	3.05	2.93	2.84	2.76	2.70	2.60	2.50	2.39	2.33	2.27	2.21	2.14	2.08	2.00
24	5.75	4.35	3.75	3.41	3.18	3.02	2.90	2.81	2.73	2.67	2.57	2.47	2.36	2.30	2.24	2.18	2.11	2.04	1.97
25	5.72	4.32	3.72	3.38	3.15	2.99	2.87	2.78	2.70	2.64	2.54	2.44	2.33	2.27	2.21	2.15	2.08	2.01	1.94
26	5.69	4.29	3.69	3.35	3.13	2.97	2.85	2.75	2.68	2.61	2.51	2.41	2.30	2.24	2.18	2.12	2.05	1.98	1.91
27	5.66	4.27	3.67	3.33	3.10	2.94	2.82	2.73	2.65	2.59	2.49	2.39	2.28	2.22	2.16	2.09	2.03	1.95	1.88
28	5.63	4.24	3.65	3.31	3.08	2.92	2.80	2.71	2.63	2.57	2.47	2.36	2.25	2.19	2.13	2.07	2.00	1.93	1.85
29	5.61	4.22	3.63	3.29	3.06	2.90	2.78	2.69	2.61	2.55	2.45	2.34	2.23	2.17	2.11	2.05	1.98	1.91	1.83
30	5.59	4.20	3.61	3.27	3.04	2.88	2.76	2.67	2.59	2.53	2.43	2.32	2.21	2.15	2.09	2.03	1.96	1.89	1.81
31	5.57	4.18	3.59	3.25	3.03	2.87	2.75	2.65	2.57	2.51	2.41	2.31	2.20	2.14	2.07	2.01	1.94	1.87	1.79
41	5.42	4.05	3.46	3.13	2.90	2.74	2.62	2.53	2.45	2.39	2.29	2.18	2.07	2.01	1.94	1.88	1.80	1.72	1.64
61	5.29	3.93	3.34	3.01	2.79	2.63	2.51	2.41	2.33	2.27	2.17	2.06	1.94	1.88	1.82	1.74	1.67	1.58	1.48
121	5.15	3.80	3.23	2.89	2.67	2.52	2.39	2.30	2.22	2.16	2.05	1.94	1.82	1.76	1.69	1.61	1.53	1.43	1.31
∞	5.02	3.69	3.12	2.79	2.57	2.41	2.29	2.19	2.11	2.05	1.94	1.83	1.71	1.64	1.57	1.48	1.39	1.27	1.00

is that standard deviations of $1.4°F$ and $0.7°F$ are in fact estimates of a common population standard deviation. This assumption is rejected by this significance test in favor of the alternative hypothesis that the standard deviations estimate different population standard deviations. This supports the contention that the patient suspected of having the condition does indeed have this illness.

Example. After a year's experience, the systolic blood pressure readings made by two graduates of a family nurse practitioner training program are compared. Although the graduates are located in different communities, it is assumed that the patient mix is the same. Since each student has been trained in a different method, it is of interest to see who has the more variable readings and whether this is significant at the 5% level. Family nurse practitioner A has a standard deviation of 24.5 mm Hg based on single blood pressure determinations in 163 different patients. Family nurse practitioner B has a standard deviation likewise of 20.0 based on 35 readings.

Clearly A has the greater variability in her blood pressure determinations. To check if this is significant at the 5% level we use a double-tailed test, since there is no a priori reason why one family nurse practitioner should have readings with higher variability than the other.

We therefore use Table 9.7b. However there is no entry for n' = 163, n'' = 35. We therefore must interpolate as follows:

$$F = \frac{(24.5)^2}{(20.0)^2} = 1.50$$

and this is lower than any of the four tabulated values in Table 9.7b adjacent to n' = 163, n'' = 35. These are:

	n' = 121	n' = ∞
n'' = 31	1.87	1.79
n'' = 41	1.72	1.64

Therefore the test is not significant. (If the calculated F value in this example had been greater than 1.87 the test would have been significant. In fact, F is less than 1.64 and so the test is non-significant. If F had fallen between 1.64 and 1.87 for n' = 163 and n'' =

35, then these tables would be inadequate and all the investigator could say is that the result is indeterminate.)

9.7 TESTS OF ASSOCIATION

The above sections have dealt exclusively with tests of significance in one continuous variable. Here we introduce tests of association between two measures and between two classifications.

9.7.1 Test of Significance of the Correlation Coefficient

The correlation coefficient r measures the strength of (linear) association between two measures in a sample. A value of $r = 0$ denotes no association, whereas $r = \pm 1$ denotes direct and inverse proportionality, respectively (apart from an additive constant). The question arises, if we find that two measures are associated with correlation coefficient r in a *sample,* whether or not the variables are associated in the population from which the sample is drawn or whether the observed value of r is just an artifact due to sampling variation. To answer this question, we use Table 9.8 to calculate the test statistic as

$$|r| = \frac{|\ \Sigma\,(x - \bar{x})\,(y - \bar{y})\ |}{\sqrt{\Sigma(x - \bar{x})^2}\ \sqrt{\Sigma(y - \bar{y})^2}}.$$

Since the correlation coefficient r may take on positive or negative values, the test is double-tailed and is considered significant if the absolute value of r, $|r|$, exceeds the tabulated value.

A rationalization of the formula for the correlation co-efficient follows:

Direct proportional association between x and y implies that y increases as x increases so that, for a large x,y will also be large and the product of xy very large. Under an inverse proportional relationship, for a large x, y will be small and the product xy relatively constant. A crude statistic of association might therefore be the average product, $\Sigma\ xy/n$. If we agree to measure from the

Table 9.8 Significance limits for $|r|$, the sample correlation coefficient

n	P 0.1	0.05	0.01	0.001	n	P 0.1	0.05	0.01	0.001
3	0.9877	0.9969	0.9999	1.0000	103	0.1630	0.1937	0.2528	0.3196
	9000	9500	9900	0.9990		1622	1927	2515	3181
	8054	8783	9587	9911		1614	1918	2504	3166
	7293	8114	9172	9741		1606	1909	2492	3152
7	0.6694	0.7545	0.8745	0.9509	107	0.1599	0.1900	0.2480	0.3138
	6215	7067	8343	9249		1591	1891	2469	3123
	5822	6664	7977	8983		1584	1882	2458	3109
	5494	6319	7646	8721		1577	1874	2447	3095
	5214	6021	7348	8471		1569	1865	2436	3082
12	0.4973	0.5760	0.7079	0.8233	112	0.1562	0.1857	0.2425	0.3069
	4762	5529	6835	8010		1555	1848	2414	3055
	4575	5324	6614	7800		1548	1840	2404	3042
	4409	5139	6411	7604		1542	1832	2393	3029
	4259	4973	6226	7419		1535	1824	2383	3017
17	0.4124	0.4821	0.6055	0.7247	117	0.1528	0.1816	0.2373	0.3004
	4000	4683	5897	7084		1522	1809	2363	2992
	3887	4555	5751	6932		1515	1801	2353	2979
	3783	4438	5614	6788		1509	1793	2343	2967
	3687	4329	5487	6652		1502	1786	2334	2955
22	0.3598	0.4227	0.5368	0.6524	122	0.1496	0.1779	0.2324	0.2943
	3515	4132	5256	6402		1490	1771	2315	2932
	3438	4044	5151	6287		1484	1764	2305	2920
	3365	3961	5052	6177		1478	1757	2296	2909
	3297	3882	4958	6073		1472	1750	2287	2897
27	0.3233	0.3809	0.4869	0.5974	127	0.1466	0.1743	0.2278	0.2886
	3172	3739	4785	5880		1460	1736	2269	2875
	3115	3673	4705	5790		1455	1730	2261	2864
	3061	3610	4629	5703		1449	1723	2252	2854
	3009	3550	4556	5620		1443	1716	2243	2843
32	0.2960	0.3494	0.4487	0.5541	132	0.1438	0.1710	0.2235	0.2832
	2913	3440	4421	5465		1432	1703	2226	2822
	2869	3388	4357	5392		1427	1697	2218	2812
	2826	3338	4297	5322		1422	1690	2210	2801
	2785	3291	4238	5255		1416	1684	2202	2791
37	0.2746	0.3246	0.4182	0.5189	137	0.1411	0.1678	0.2194	0.2781
	2709	3202	4128	5126		1406	1672	2186	2771
	2673	3160	4076	5066		1401	1666	2178	2762
	2638	3120	4026	5007		1396	1660	2170	2752
	2605	3081	3978	4951		1391	1654	2163	2742
42	0.2573	0.3044	0.3932	0.4896	142	0.1386	0.1648	0.2155	0.2733
	2542	3008	3887	4843		1381	1642	2148	2724
	2512	2973	3843	4792		1376	1637	2140	2714
	2483	2940	3802	4742		1371	1631	2133	2705
	2455	2907	3761	4694		1367	1625	2126	2696
47	0.2428	0.2875	0.3721	0.4647	147	0.1362	0.1620	0.2118	0.2687
	2403	2845	3683	4602		1357	1614	2111	2678
	2377	2816	3646	4558		1353	1609	2104	2669
	2353	2787	3610	4515		1348	1603	2097	2660
	2329	2759	3575	4473		1344	1598	2090	2652
52	0.2306	0.2732	0.3541	0.4433	152	0.1339	0.1593	0.2083	0.2643
	2284	2706	3509	4393		1335	1587	2077	2635
	2262	2681	3477	4355		1330	1582	2070	2626
	2241	2656	3445	4317		1326	1577	2063	2618
	2221	2632	3415	4281		1322	1572	2057	2610
57	0.2201	0.2609	0.3385	0.4245	157	0.1318	0.1567	0.2050	0.2602
	2181	2586	3357	4210		1313	1562	2044	2594
	2162	2564	3329	4176		1309	1557	2037	2586
	2144	2542	3301	4143		1305	1552	2031	2578
	2126	2521	3274	4111		1301	1547	2025	2570
62	0.2108	0.2500	0.3248	0.4079	162	0.1297	0.1543	0.2019	0.2562
	2091	2480	3223	4048		1293	1538	2012	2554
	2075	2461	3198	4018		1289	1533	2006	2547
	2058	2442	3174	3988		1285	1529	2000	2539
	2042	2423	3150	3959		1281	1524	1994	2532
67	0.2027	0.2405	0.3127	0.3931	167	0.1277	0.1519	0.1988	0.2524
	2012	2387	3104	3904		1273	1515	1982	2517
	1997	2369	3081	3877		1270	1510	1977	2510
	1982	2352	3060	3850		1266	1506	1971	2502
	1968	2335	3038	3824		1262	1501	1965	2495
72	0.1954	0.2319	0.3017	0.3798	172	0.1258	0.1497	0.1959	0.2488
	1940	2303	2997	3773		1255	1493	1954	2481
	1927	2287	2977	3749		1251	1488	1948	2474
	1914	2272	2957	3725		1248	1484	1943	2467
	1901	2257	2938	3701		1244	1480	1937	2460
77	0.1889	0.2242	0.2919	0.3678	177	0.1240	0.1476	0.1932	0.2453
	1876	2227	2900	3655		1237	1471	1926	2446
	1864	2213	2882	3633		1233	1467	1921	2440
	1852	2199	2864	3611		1230	1463	1915	2433
	1841	2185	2847	3590		1227	1459	1910	2426
82	0.1829	0.2172	0.2830	0.3569	182	0.1223	0.1455	0.1905	0.2420
	1818	2159	2813	3548		1220	1451	1900	2413
	1807	2146	2796	3527		1216	1447	1895	2407
	1796	2133	2780	3507		1213	1443	1890	2400
	1786	2120	2764	3488		1210	1439	1885	2394
87	0.1775	0.2108	0.2748	0.3468	187	0.1207	0.1435	0.1880	0.2388
	1765	2096	2733	3449		1203	1432	1874	2381
	1755	2084	2717	3430		1200	1428	1870	2375
	1745	2072	2702	3412		1197	1424	1865	2369
	1735	2061	2688	3394		1194	1420	1860	2363
92	0.1726	0.2050	0.2673	0.3376	192	0.1191	0.1417	0.1855	0.2357
	1716	2039	2659	3358		1188	1413	1850	2351
	1707	2028	2645	3341		1184	1409	1845	2345
	1698	2017	2631	3324		1181	1406	1841	2339
	1689	2006	2617	3307		1178	1402	1836	2333
97	0.1680	0.1996	0.2604	0.3291	197	0.1175	0.1399	0.1831	0.2327
	1671	1986	2591	3274		1172	1395	1827	2321
	1663	1976	2578	3258		1169	1391	1822	2316
	1654	1966	2565	3242		1166	1388	1818	2310
	1646	1956	2552	3227		1164	1384	1813	2304
102	0.1638	0.1946	0.2540	0.3211	202	0.1161	0.1381	0.1809	0.2299

From *Documenta Geigy Scientific Tables,* 7th ed., 1971, p. 61, by permission of the publishers Ciba-Geigy Ltd., Basel, Switzerland.

double mean $(\bar{x}, \bar{y})$ then this expression becomes $\Sigma\ (x-\bar{x})(y-\bar{y})/n$. Now if x and y are in fact independent this product will be zero, giving us a reference standard, i.e., two truly independent measures will yield a zero correlation coefficient. Finally, if we have a perfect association so that in fact x and y are identical the statistic will become $\Sigma\ (x-\bar{x})(x-\bar{x})/n$. Hence if we divide $\Sigma\ (x-\bar{x})(y-\bar{y})/n$ by $\Sigma\ (x-\bar{x})^2/n$ the statistic will take value 1 for perfect correlation. Since we could equally well substitute x for y we could also justify dividing by $\Sigma\ (y-\bar{y})/n$. In fact we compromise by dividing $\Sigma\ (x-\bar{x})(y-\bar{y})/n$ by the square root of the product of $\Sigma\ (x-\bar{x})^2/n$ and $\Sigma\ (y-\bar{y})^2/n$ to get

$$r = \frac{\Sigma\ (x-\bar{x})(y-\bar{y})}{\sqrt{\Sigma\ (x-\bar{x})^2}\ \sqrt{\Sigma\ (y-\bar{y})^2}}$$

since the sample size cancels. An alternative justification of the expression for the correlation coefficient is to recognize it as $\Sigma x'y'$ where x', y' are normalized transformations of x, y, i.e.:

$$x' = \frac{x-\bar{x}}{s_x}$$

$$y' = \frac{y-\bar{y}}{s_y}$$

Example. Over the past few years, records have been kept of the mean waiting time of outpatients in an emergency clinic and of the total number of attending physicians and nurses. Before deciding whether to reduce or increase the number of people on the staff serving the clinic, a correlation coefficient is calculated from the data to confirm that waiting time changes as the number of professionals increases. In all, 72 pairs of observations were available and gave a correlation coefficient of -0.298. From Table 9.8, with $n = 72$, we find that 0.298 falls between the tabulated values associated with 5% and 1% probability. Therefore, we can state that this correlation coefficient is significant (meaning significantly different from zero) $(0.05 > P > 0.01)$ and we must reject the implied assumption that there was no association between staff size and waiting time in the emergency clinic.

Now if we wish to calculate the increase in mean waiting time caused by a decrease in the staff of one member, we can use the

regression equation associated with this correlation coefficient of
−0.298, knowing that the regression equation will be based on a
significant relationship between staff size and waiting time. However, since r^2 is equal to the proportion of variation explained by
the relationship, we should not depend too heavily on this relationship in the future, since only 9% of future variation is affected
by staffing levels.

9.7.2 χ^2-Statistic: Testing of Association among Classifications and Tests of Differences between Proportions

In the immediately preceding example, we treated the number of
professionals as a measure although we know that in fact this is a
count. We can do this because of the large number of classes in the
count, and the presumed approximation of its distribution to the
normal distribution.

　　Most classifications, however, do not contain many classes and
do not have any underlying ranking of the classes. To test for
association among such classifications we use the χ^2 statistic,
which is tabulated in Table 9.9. The test used is

$$\chi^2 = \sum \frac{(O - E)^2}{E}$$

where

O = the number falling into a given cell of a table,
E = expected number for that cell,
Σ = the sum over all cells of the table.

In the χ^2-test for association, the expected number E is calculated
as the product of the row and column totals for that cell divided
by the grand total.

Example. A dentist wishes to test whether there is an association
between eye color and sensitivity to oral pain. He classifies 60 of
his patients according to these classifications and derives the
"observed" table. From the row and column totals of the "observed" table, he then calculates the "expected" table. These are
shown in Table 9.10.

Table 9.9. Significance limits for χ^2 calculated from a table with ν degrees of freedom (see Section 9.7.2)

	P			P	
ν	0.050	0.010	ν	0.050	0.010
1	3.841	6.635	51	68.669	77.386
2	5.991	9.210	52	69.832	78.616
3	7.815	11.345	53	70.993	79.843
4	9.488	13.277	54	72.153	81.069
5	11.070	15.086	55	73.311	82.292
6	12.592	16.812	56	74.468	83.513
7	14.067	18.475	57	75.624	84.733
8	15.507	20.090	58	76.778	85.950
9	16.919	21.666	59	77.931	87.166
10	18.307	23.209	60	79.082	88.379
11	19.675	24.725	61	80.232	89.591
12	21.026	26.217	62	81.381	90.802
13	22.362	27.688	63	82.529	92.010
14	23.685	29.141	64	83.675	93.217
15	24.996	30.578	65	84.821	94.422
16	26.296	32.000	66	85.965	95.626
17	27.587	33.409	67	87.108	96.828
18	28.869	34.805	68	88.250	98.028
19	30.144	36.191	69	89.391	99.227
20	31.410	37.566	70	90.531	100.425
21	32.671	38.932	71	91.670	101.621
22	33.924	40.289	72	92.808	102.816
23	35.172	41.638	73	93.945	104.010
24	36.415	42.980	74	95.081	105.202
25	37.652	44.314	75	96.217	106.393
26	38.885	45.642	76	97.351	107.583
27	40.113	46.963	77	98.484	108.771
28	41.337	48.278	78	99.617	109.958
29	42.557	49.588	79	100.749	111.144
30	43.773	50.892	80	101.879	112.329
31	44.985	52.191	81	103.009	113.512
32	46.194	53.486	82	104.139	114.695
33	47.400	54.776	83	105.267	115.876
34	48.602	56.061	84	106.395	117.057
35	49.802	57.342	85	107.522	118.236
36	50.998	58.619	86	108.648	119.414
37	52.192	59.892	87	109.773	120.591
38	53.384	61.162	88	110.898	121.767
39	54.572	62.428	89	112.022	122.942
40	55.758	63.691	90	113.145	124.116
41	56.942	64.950	91	114.268	125.289
42	58.124	66.206	92	115.390	126.462
43	59.304	67.459	93	116.511	127.633
44	60.481	68.709	94	117.632	128.803
45	61.656	69.957	95	118.752	129.973
46	.62.830	71.201	96	119.871	131.141
47	64.001	72.443	97	120.990	132.309
48	65.171	73.683	98	122.108	133.476
49	66.339	74.919	99	123.225	134.642
50	67.505	76.154	100	124.342	135.806

From *Documenta Geigy Scientific Tables,* 7th ed., 1971, pp. 36-37, by permission of the publishers Ciba-Geigy Ltd., Basel, Switzerland.

Table 9.10. Observed and expected frequencies

Table of "observed" frequencies

Eye color	Sensitivity to oral pain			Total
	High	Moderate	Low	
Blue	10	6	4	20
Brown	5	10	15	30
Gray	0	4	6	10
Total	15	20	25	60

Table of "expected" frequencies

Eye color	Sensitivity to oral pain			Total
	High	Moderate	Low	
Blue	$15 \times 20/60 = 5.0$	$20 \times 20/60 = 6.7$	$20 - 5.0 - 6.7 = 8.3$	20
Brown	$15 \times 30/60 = 7.5$	$20 \times 30/60 = 10.0$	$30 - 7.5 - 10.0 = 12.5$	30
Gray	$15 - 5.0 - 7.5 = 2.5$	$20 - 6.7 - 10.0 = 3.3$	$25 - 8.3 - 12.5 = 4.2$	10
Total	15	20	25	60

The χ^2 value evaluated on this sample of 60 patients is then

$$\chi^2 = \frac{(10-5.0)^2}{5.0} + \frac{(6-6.7)^2}{6.7} + \frac{(4-8.3)^2}{8.3}$$

$$+ \frac{(5-7.5)^2}{7.5} + \frac{(10-10.0)^2}{10.0} + \frac{(15-12.5)^2}{12.5}$$

$$+ \frac{(0-2.5)^2}{2.5} + \frac{(4-3.3)^2}{3.3} + \frac{(6-4.2)^2}{4.2}$$

$$= 12.05.$$

The value of χ^2 associated with a probability of 5% is obtained from Table 9.9, entering this table with the number v calculated as

$$v = (\text{number of rows} - 1) \times (\text{number of columns} - 1).$$

In this example, $v = 2 \times 2 = 4$. (Note that given the row and column totals, we need to calculate only the expected values for v = 4 cells. The expected values in the remaining 5 cells can be obtained by subtracting from the row and column totals. See the table of expected values in Table 9.10.)

The χ^2 value for $\nu = 4$ and $P = 0.05$ from Table 9.9 is equal to 9.488. The calculated value of χ^2 is greater than this and, therefore, we reject the assumption that eye color and sensitivity to oral pain are independent. (To see how they are associated, compare the relative sizes of the observed and expected values in the cells of the table. This suggests that patients with blue eyes are more likely to have a high sensitivity to oral pain than patients with brown or gray eyes.)

Note that the χ^2 test is based on the number observed and expected in the cells of a given two-way table. χ^2 is applicable only to test the independence of two classifications (not measures) given the two-way *frequency* table for these classifications.

The χ^2 test of significance may also be used to test whether the frequency distributions in two samples are significantly different. The most common form of this test is the test of the difference of two proportions from two different samples. This test is carried out as above. (There are other approaches, however, including alternative formulations and tables for direct evaluation of the difference when the sample sizes are small. The reader is referred to other texts for these. For a comprehensive treatment of the analysis of classifications see Maxwell, 1961.)

Example. A sample was taken of the hospitals in each of two adjoining states. In each sample the percentage of hospitals in which the chief hospital administrator had an M.D. degree was recorded. In the more northern state, 15% (9 out of 60) of the sampled hospital directors had M.D.'s, whereas in the more southern state, 20% (16 out of 80) had this degree. Test whether there is a significant difference at the 5% level between these two percentages.

Table 9.11 gives the observed and expected distributions of directors' qualifications by state. Note that in the table of expected values there is only one cell that can be arbitrarily specified so that $\nu = 1$. Applying the formula, we get

$$\nu = (\text{number of rows} - 1) \times (\text{number of columns} - 1)$$

$$= (2 - 1) \times (2 - 1) = 1.$$

Table 9.11. Observed and expected distributions

Observed distribution

| | Qualifications of hospital directors | | |
	M.D.'s	Other	Total
More northern state	9	51	60
More southern state	16	64	80
Total	25	115	140

Expected distribution

| | Qualifications of hospital directors | | |
	M.D.'s	Other	Total
More northern state	25 × 60/140 = 10.7	60 - 10.7 = 49.3	60
More southern state	25 - 10.7 = 14.3	80 - 14.3 = 65.7	80
Total	25	115	140

The 5% tabulated χ^2 value for $\nu = 1$ is 3.841. The value of the χ^2 test statistic calculated from the sample is

$$\chi^2 = \frac{(9 - 10.7)^2}{10.7} + \frac{(51 - 49.3)^2}{49.3} + \frac{(16 - 14.3)^2}{14.3} + \frac{(64 - 65.7)^2}{65.7}$$

$$= 0.57.$$

Since the calculated value of χ^2 is less than the 5% tabulated value, the test is not significant and we retain the original assumption from which the expected values were calculated, namely, that the two sample proportions both estimate the same common population proportion. We conclude that there is insufficient evidence in this information to reject the assumption that the more northern state and the more southern state employ the same proportion of hospital directors with M.D. degrees.

EXERCISES

9.1 "Statistics cannot prove anything." Comment on this statement and illustrate your reply by referring to significance levels.

9.2 Nineteen independent tests of saliva have a mean of 7.6 pH units and a range of 2.4 pH units. Using Table 9.1,
  a) test whether this sample mean is significantly different from a "true" pH level of 7.0 pH units (at the 5% level of significance),
  b) from a "true" pH level of 7.9 pH units,
  c) from a "true" pH level of 7.45 pH units,
  d) state your assumptions in using Table 9.1.

9.3 The sample size in Exercise 9.2 is changed to 28. The mean and standard deviation in this sample are now 7.5 ± 1.1. Using Table 9.2,
  a) test whether the sample mean of 7.5 is significantly different from a "true" mean of 7.0,
  b) test whether the sample mean of 7.5 is significantly different from a "true" mean of 7.8,
  c) state how the assumptions made in using Table 9.2 differ from those in Exercise 9.2 using Table 9.1 (if at all).

9.4 The sample size in Exercise 9.2 is increased to 103. The mean and standard deviation of the pH level measure in the (large) sample of 103 is 7.23 ± 1.33 pH units. Using Table 9.3,
  a) test whether the sample mean of 7.23 is significantly different (at the 5% level) from a "true" mean of 7.0 pH units,
  b) test whether this mean is significantly different from a "true" mean of 7.50,
  c) state what assumptions are necessary in using Table 9.3 in this problem.

9.5 The direct nursing costs per patient for two intensive care units of a large university hospital are compared by an industrial engineer. He selects 14 days at random in the past quarter and calculates for each of these days the direct nursing costs per patient in each of the two units. He summarizes his results as shown in the following table:

Direct Nursing Costs per Patient

	Respiratory unit	Cardiac unit
Number of days sampled	14	14
Mean	$33.20	$39.79
Maximum	$63.14	$58.70
Minimum	$25.60	$32.80

  a) Using Table 9.4, test whether at the 5% level of significance there is a difference in the mean direct nursing costs per patient per day between the two intensive care units in the quarter.
  b) What assumptions are made in using Table 9.4 in answering this problem?

9.6 In Exercise 9.5, the 14 observations for the cardiac unit are ranked in increasing order of size.

a) Using the 5% level of significance, test the hypothesis that the quarter's daily direct nursing costs are normally distributed given that

$$x_{(1)} = 32.80, \quad x_{(2)} = 33.50, \quad x_{(3)} = 35.21,$$

$$x_{(14)} = 58.70, \quad x_{(13)} = 51.42, \quad x_{(12)} = 48.16.$$

b) What assumptions are made in using Table 9.5 for this test?

9.7 A patient's temperature is taken night and morning for three days. The chart shows the following values in the order in which they were taken:

$$102.6, \quad 98.6, \quad 102.0, \quad 99.0, \quad 101.8, \quad 99.0.$$

Test whether at the 10% level of significance we can assume that the patient's "true" temperature is free from nonrandom influences such a diurnal cycles or a trend over time.

9.8 In Exercise 9.5 the standard deviations of the two samples, each of size 14, were calculated. These were $6.25 and $4.00 for the respiratory and cardiac intensive care units, respectively. Using Table 9.7 test at the 5% level whether there is a significant difference in the variation of direct nursing costs per patient from day to day in the two units.

9.9 From information provided by the Hospitals Administration Services program, the regression equation between y = percent of total annual hospital expenses devoted to nursing services and x = number of hospital beds is given as

$$\hat{y} = 31 - 0.02x,$$

where $\hat{y}$ is the value of y predicted by the regression equation for a given number of beds x. If this regression equation is calculated from data on 162 participating hospitals and if

   s_x = sample standard deviation of the number of beds
       = 51,

and

   s_y = sample standard deviation of the percent of total
       expenses for nursing
       = 8,

test whether, at the 5% level, the regression equation is "significant." (*Hint:* Test whether the regression coefficient (-0.02) is significantly different from zero. Convert -0.02 to its equivalent correlation coefficient using the relation

$$r = b \frac{s_x}{s_y}$$

and use Table 9.8 to test the "significance" of r, i.e., whether the associated correlation coefficient is significantly different from zero. If it is, then the regression equation may be of value in prediction.)

9.10 Omitting the three sublingual tumors in Table 2.3, test whether there is a significant difference (at the 5% level) between the frequency of parotid tumors that are malignant and the frequency of submaxillary tumors that are malignant. (*Hint:* Form a 2 × 2 table and calculate χ^2 to be evaluated in Table 9.9.)

9.11 Assuming that in Figure 2.8 each of the three age groups contained 100 individuals, test by means of χ^2 whether there is a significant relationship between age group and type of accident and describe it if it is significant. (*Hint:* It will be necessary to round off the given percentages in such a manner that they are counts which add up to 100.)

9.12 From Exercise 7.3, form a 2 × 2 table and use χ^2 to test the significance of the difference between the proportion of blacks employed and hospitalized.

LITERATURE CITED

Feinberg, W. E. 1971. Teaching the Type I and Type II Errors: The Judicial Process. Amer. Statis. 25(3):30–32.

Maxwell, A. E. 1961. Analysing Qualitative Data. Methuen & Co. Ltd., London.

Shafer, W. G., M. K. Hine, and B. M. Levy. 1963. A Textbook of Oral Pathology. 2nd Ed. W. B. Saunders Company, Philadelphia.

Snedecor, G. W., and W. F. Cochran. 1967. Statistical Methods. 6th Ed. Iowa State University Press, Ames, Iowa.

10
Decisions in Health Care

10.1 INTRODUCTION

The emphasis of this text is on applications of classical statistical principles to observations in health care research and administration. Thus, in the preceding chapters, we have emphasized statistical inference and tests of significance. In the following pages, we attempt to describe briefly some of the applications of statistics to decision making. As will be seen (and as recommended by a task force on quantitative methods in hospital administration [Griffith, 1970]), the material in the first six chapters of this text is necessary for an appreciation of the procedures described below. In the next section we introduce the **cost function** approach, in which the future benefits and costs for a given decision are compared. In this approach these costs and benefits are measured in financial terms. Since not all benefits and costs can be measured or evaluated in terms of money, we introduce the concept of personal **utility** to cover the many situations in health care where ethical and humanitarian concepts have to be included. The formal structure of decision making is introduced and is illustrated by a hypothetical example. A more formal treatment of decision making is given by Raiffa (1968). The chapter concludes with considerations of **control charts** for both continuous and discrete variables and with examples of their application to health problems.

10.2 COST FUNCTIONS

Consider the following situation. An insurance company offers benefits of $20 for each full day the insured spends in the hospital. The premium is $5 per month (for individuals aged between 15 and 44 years who have never been refused health insurance or coverage). Hospitalization for conditions existing before the insurance takes effect will not be paid for during the first two years of the coverage. How does an individual arrive at the decision to insure himself or not to insure himself under the plan?

One of the first principles of decision theory is that decisions are made rationally to maximize the expected return. An individual might make a decision to insure himself or not (assuming he was eligible) by reasoning that in one year he will pay $60 in premiums and will recoup this amount if he spends three days in the hospital with benefits of $20 per day. Next, in deciding whether to participate, he will probably use a combination of past information and his desire for this type of hospital coverage in the future. If he believes he will not need this coverage next year he will not insure himself. However, if he thinks that he is likely to spend three or more days in the hospital, he would be inclined to insure himself. The great majority of people, however, will make a decision on this type of coverage depending on their current assets and desire for insurance in the future. (Decisions made on the basis of **expected** utility are described in the next section.)

The cost-function approach to decision making is similar to this in philosophy but a little more elaborate, and it involves the use of probabilities. A cost-function approach contrasts expected costs with expected benefits, and a decision is made according to which is greater. In the above situation, the expected cost of premiums in the year is $60. We know this with certainty, assuming that the insured stays in the scheme one year and that rates do not change. The expected benefits are $20 times the expected number of days in the hospital in one year. The expected number of days a person will be hospitalized is given by the expression

$$\sum_{i=1}^{365} iP_i = 0P_0 + 1P_1 + 2P_2 + 3P_3 + \ldots ,$$

where i = a given number of hospitalized days 0, 1, 2, . . . , 365 and P_i = the probability of spending a total of i days in the hospital that year. This expression is the same as that used to calculate a mean from a frequency distribution (see Exercise 5.1):

$$\bar{x} = 0f_0 + 1f_1 + 2f_2 + 3f_3 + \cdots$$

In both cases, the probabilities and the relative frequencies add up to 1.

The next question is where do the values of P_i come from? Since these are future probabilities for that individual, they cannot be known. We could, however, use past information for this individual, forming a frequency distribution of the number of days of hospitalization per year over his lifetime to date. This assumes that next year's experience will be a random sample of one observation from this frequency distribution. The number of observations in this distribution will, however, be small, being equal to the person's age. Also, the use of this distribution assumes erroneously that the probability of hospitalization remains constant despite one's age. An alternative approach is to use last year's frequency distribution for all individuals of comparable age. While this frequency distribution will be based on many observations, in using it we shall have to assume that the individual is average or typical in his hospitalization experience and that the distribution will describe his probabilities of hospitalization for zero, one, two, three, or more days in the coming year.

Assume for the sake of illustration that the distribution is as shown in Table 10.1. Then the expected or mean number of days spent in the hospital by a randomly selected member of this population last year is

$$0.15 \times 1 + 0.20 \times 2 + 0.05 \times 3 + 0.03 \times 5 + 0.01 \times 16.5$$
$$+ 0.02 \times 37.5 + 0.01 \times 72.5 + 0.01 \times 142.5 = 3.915$$

and if this distribution is applicable next year to this individual, his expected return would be

$$\$20 \times 3.915 = \$78.30.$$

Since the expected benefits are greater than the expected costs, the decision to insure would follow.

In the above, we have omitted any considerations of the

Table 10.1. Hypothetical distribution of stay in hospitals for 34-year-old males earning $10,000–$14,999 per annum

Stay in hospital	Frequency (per cent)	Midpoint (days)
0 days	52	0
1 day	15	1
2 days	20	2
3 days	5	3
4–6 days	3	5
1–3 weeks	1	16.5
4–6 weeks	2	37.5
7–13 weeks	1	72.5
14–26 weeks	1	142.5
27–39 weeks	0	233.5
40–52 weeks	0	324.5
	100	

interest on $60 saved at the rate of $5 per month over a year. Also, we have used the net amount of money expected to be gained as the sole criterion for the decision. Other considerations, such as the need to continue a minimum income for one's dependents while in the hospital, are important in deciding whether or not to insure oneself. These criticisms call for a more inclusive criterion such as utility, as outlined below. (The above calculation cannot be realistic, since the company would lose money insuring 34-year-old males in this income bracket!)

10.3   UTILITIES AND DECISION MAKING

10.3.1   Utilities

Consider the following hypothetical situation. The director of an understaffed 100-bed hospital is considering removing a number of beds because of an acute nursing shortage. He is concerned with two conflicting criteria: morale of the nursing staff and the public's need for hospitalization. He can attempt to measure these criteria with indices ranging from 0 to 1. Zero will represent the low point of the scale and 1 the high point, and he desires to maximize these indices by his actions, i.e., to compromise in the number of beds to remove, since nurse morale improves but public service declines as the number of beds decreases (over the range he is considering).

The director considers taking multiples of 10 beds out of service and draws up a table such as Table 10.2 to guide him to the best choice. In this table, he tries to quantify the result of removing 10 or more beds in terms of the change in the indices of staff morale and public service. He also sets down the relative **weights** he would give to these indices for each decision. With this subjective quantification, he can then combine the two indices with their relative weights to get a value of the utility of each decision. Because of its definition, the utility scale ranges from 0 to 1. If we choose that decision that maximized the utility, the director would remove 10 beds. However, he should remember that these figures are guesses and try to refine them at least in the region of the optimal decision, say, from 0 to 20 beds (since the utility over this region varies from 0.85 to 0.82 with a maximum of 0.86 for a reduction of 10 beds).

This hypothetical example illustrates the concept of utilities, when decisions must be evaluated in terms of multiple conse- quences that cannot be measured in dollars. A more formal defini- tion is couched in terms of the equivalence of a given utility to a lottery with a stated chance or probability of winning a desirable prize (Raiffa, 1968, p. 57). The relative weighting given by the hospital director in Table 10.2 to pairs of values of indices for morale and public service reflects the fact that he does not consider a constant equivalence between the two indices at dif- ferent levels in bed reduction. Note also that over the range of 0 to 20 beds removed the expected utility is approximately a constant. (Actually it ranges from 0.86 to 0.82.) This would suggest that, over this range, there might be a constant equivalence between the two indices. This means that a reduction of one unit in one index would be acceptable if the increase in the other index were λ units, where λ is the **substitution constant**.

10.3.2 Decision Theory

To illustrate the structure of decision making, we revert to a situation in which the consequences are measured in dollars.

Table 10.2. Choices of number of beds to close

Number of beds removed	Number remaining	Staff morale index	Public service index	Relative weights		Expected utility
0	100	0.70	1.00	0.50	0.50	0.35 + 0.50 = 0.85
10	90	0.80	0.90	0.40	0.60	0.32 + 0.54 = 0.86
20	80	0.85	0.80	0.35	0.65	0.30 + 0.52 = 0.82
30	70	0.90	0.70	0.30	0.70	0.27 + 0.49 = 0.76
40	60	1.00	0.60	0.30	0.70	0.30 + 0.42 = 0.72
50	50	0.95	0.50	0.30	0.70	0.29 + 0.34 = 0.63
60	40	0.80	0.40	0.25	0.75	0.20 + 0.30 = 0.50
70	30	0.50	0.30	0.40	0.60	0.20 + 0.18 = 0.38

Assume that a former patient owes the hospital $1,000. A number of options are possible in trying to recover the debt. Assume that these can only be successful or unsuccessful, i.e., that partial repayment of the debt is not possible. The options, by increasing cost, are to write off (W.O.) the whole debt, to write a letter (L), to call in a debt collection agency (D), or to go to court (C). The probabilities of success and costs of these options are as shown in Table 10.3. Further, to simplify the illustration, let us assume that if a letter fails we would not go to court before trying to collect the debt through an agency, but we may decide to write off the debt at any time.

To show the **decision tree,** we introduce the convention of a square box to represent a time at which a decision is made and a circle for a time at which a response occurs over which the decision maker has no influence. The circle may be considered a time at which a raffle is drawn to determine which of several consequences occurs following a certain course of action. The decision tree is shown in Figure 10.1. Note that the squares are numbered for ease of reference to the figure. Consider the lowest line, marked C. This represents the decision to go to court. The circle at the end of this line represents the trial at which (hypothetically) the hospital has a 50% chance of being awarded $1,000 and a 50% chance of losing the trial and getting nothing. The expected return at the beginning of the trial is, therefore, 0.5 × $1,000 + 0.50 × $0 = $500. However, the cost of the trial to the hospital is $150 irrespective of the outcome, so the net expected return at the beginning of the trial is only $350 (i.e., $500 − $150). Note that the circle representing the chance event of trial

Table 10.3. Choices in recovering a debt

Option	P(success)	Cost
Court (C)	0.50	$150
Debt collection (D)	0.10	10
Letter (L)	0.01	1
Write off (W.O.)	0.00	0

Figure 10.1. Decision tree.

182

has inscribed in it the cost of the trial (−$150) and has the net expected return ($350) printed above the circle.

The decision to employ a debt collection agency (D) to recover $1,000 owed is shown by the lowest line marked D. To trace this path, we note that the debt collection will be either successful (and, by assumption, recover $1,000) or will fail. If this strategy fails, then by our rules, the hospital director can either write off the debt or go to court with, as shown above, an expected net return of $350. If he chooses the first alternative and writes off the debt, his expected return is $0, so he should take the decision to go to court. Two lines are drawn across the write off line (marked W.O.) to indicate that at decision point 3 his optimal strategy is to go to court. The expected net return ($350) of the optimal path is printed above the **decision point** for later use. Now we calculate the expected net return at the chance point between 1 and 3. This forks into two possible responses: either the agency collects the $1,000 with probability 0.1 or it does not (with probability 0.9). The expected value at this **chance point**, therefore, is:

$$0.1 \times \$1,000 + 0.9 \times \$350 = \$415.$$

Here the $350 represents the maximum net expected return if the debt collection fails and the decision maker follows the best strategy (i.e., goes to court). From the expected return of $415 at this chance point the cost of the debt collection ($10) must be subtracted to give a net expected return of $405. This is printed above the chance point.

The decision path that represents sending a letter (L) demanding repayment of the debt is similarly constructed. If the letter fails (for which the probability is 0.99), then the decision maker has three choices: to write off the debt (W.O.) with zero expectation, to call in a debt collector (D) with an expectation of $405, or to go to court (C) with an expected net return of $350. Since the D path gives the highest expectation, this is selected and the other two are blocked out. The maximum dollar value at 2 is, therefore, $405. The chance point between 1 and 2 has, therefore, an expected value of

$$0.01 \times \$1,000 + 0.99 \times \$405 = \$10 + \$401 = \$411.$$

From this we subtract the cost of a letter to get a net expected value of $410. Since we know that the W.O. path has zero expectation, we can now evaluate the four initial options, W.O., L, D, and C. Of these, L has highest monetary expectation ($410) with D second ($405) and C third ($350). Therefore, we follow the optimal route along the L path, which means that to maximize our return we first send a letter, then call in a debt collection service, and finally go to court.

The reader may object to the values attached to the costs and probabilities of success, but the point is that even with crude estimates, we arrive at a set of decisions that would probably be chosen by a decision maker "flying by the seat of his pants." One could refine this formulation by allowing for legal appeals if the court case fails, by repeated efforts by debt-collecting agencies, and by repeated letters. Also, the artificial assumption of an all-or-nothing return could be replaced by enumerating different degrees of debt settlement with their associated probabilities.

The process of decision-making as outlined above may be summarized in the following four stages:

Stage 1. Outline the structure of the decision problem, enumerating the alternatives, and separating the decision points from the chance points.

Stage 2. Determine the terminal monetary rewards or utilities to be gained and the costs of the alternative options.

Stage 3. Determine the probabilities of all chance outcomes, i.e., outside the control of the decision maker.

Stage 4. Calculate, from end to beginning, the net expected value at each choice point and selecting the one option leading to the maximum value.

If a fifth stage were to be added, it would be to consider the result, in the light of your previous expectation of the result, and to check the above four stages, possibly altering and refining your definition of the problem.

10.4   QUALITY CONTROL AND NORMAL VALUES

A control chart is a graph of a repeatedly sampled statistic over time on which control limits have been drawn. These limits are based on a knowledge of the sampling distribution of the statistic graphed. A system is said to be "in control" as long as the sample statistic falls within these limits. Values can fall outside control limits for a number of reasons but, when this happens, it is generally assumed that the parameters of the system have changed, requiring intervention to bring the system back into "control."

Control limits that are too far apart will permit one falsely to conclude that the system has not changed. On the other hand, limits that are too close together will lead to intervention when this is unnecessary. A considerable literature is available on quality control and control charts, mostly in industrial settings. These texts on quality control and charting give tables by which control limits can be drawn for the different types of charts. These limits are chosen to have the desired properties with regard to both types of error.

Control charts may be used either to chart the tolerance limits of a repeatedly sampled (and possibly changing) population or to ensure that the average product of some system is unchanged. We briefly review the application of control charts to normal limits before considering the more common use of control charts in quality control.

According to Mainland (1968, p. 20) "charts or tables are often used to display trends in hospitals." While control charts were developed for the maintenance of quality in manufacturer's production lines, the health professions use a similar technique in their concept of a normal range of variation for healthy individuals. In this context, the word "normal" does not apply to the normal distribution. Control charts and normal ranges, although similar in their philosophy, refer to different things. The **normal range** of variation for blood pressure, say, is concerned with judging whether an individual falls within or outside normal limits, whereas a control chart is used to find out whether the process has gone out of control, i.e., whether the population mean has changed.

In the case of a normal range of values, such as blood pressure, where the measure approximately follows a normal distribution, the normal range is often defined as

$$\mu \pm 2\sigma,$$

which contains about 95% of the population. Note that μ and σ are the population mean and standard deviation, which are known either because the whole population has been examined (which is unlikely) or because a large random sample of the population has given estimates that may be treated as error-free. Reference to some of the original sources for normal values, however, reveals that many are based on a small number of observations from individuals who happened to be accessible to the investigator, i.e., not in any sense a random sample of the population. The statistician cannot allow for unknown bias, but he can adjust for small sample estimates by using constants given in Table 10.4 to calculate more accurately the normal range, i.e., limits that will cut off 95% of a (normally distributed) population. Thus, for example, *Documenta Geigy Scientific Tables* (1962, p. 597) gives the 95% range of values for potassium (mg/100 ml) in cerebrospinal fluid, based on 20 healthy subjects, to be 8.05 to 15.09. Since the mean is given as 11.57 and the standard deviation as 1.76, these limits are derived from $11.57 \pm 2 \times 1.76$. Reference to Table 10.4 shows that, given the sample size, the sample mean, and sample deviation, the calculation should be:

$$\bar{x} \pm cs = 11.57 \pm 2.14 \times 1.76 = 11.57 \pm 3.77 = 7.80 \text{ to } 15.34,$$

where c is a constant derived from the table.

We return now to the traditional viewpoint of quality control. The more conventional application of control charting involves the use of the standard error so that the limits are, in effect, the confidence limits

$$\mu \pm 2\sigma_{\bar{x}} \quad \text{or} \quad \mathcal{P} \pm 2\sigma_p.$$

These limits are approximate for sample means and proportions and are expressed in terms of population parameters where

$\sigma_{\bar{x}}$ represents the standard error of the sampling distribution of repeated sample means $\bar{x}$ from samples of given size about μ, and

Table 10.4. Values of c such that $\bar{x} \pm$ cs will contain 95% and 99% of the population when $\bar{x}$ and s are determined from a sample of size n randomly chosen from a normally distributed population

n	95%	99%	n	95%	99%
2	15.562	77.964	51	0282	7039
3	4.9683	11.460	52	0269	7014
4	3.5581	6.5303	53	0255	6989
5	3.0414	5.0435	54	0243	6965
6	2.7766	4.3552	55	2.0230	2.6942
7	2.6158	3.9634	56	0219	6920
8	2.5080	3.7118	57	0208	6899
9	2.4307	3.5369	58	0197	6878
10	2.3726	3.4084	59	0186	6858
11	3272	3.3102	60	2.0176	2.6839
12	2909	3.2326	61	0166	6820
13	2610	3.1698	62	0157	6803
14	2362	3.1180	63	0148	6785
15	2.2151	3.0744	64	0139	6769
16	1971	3.0374	65	2.0130	2.6753
17	1814	3.0055	66	0122	6737
18	1676	2.9776	67	0114	6722
19	1555	2.9532	68	0107	6707
20	2.1447	2.9315	69	0099	6692
21	1351	9123	70	2.0092	2.6679
22	1263	8950	71	0085	6666
23	1185	8794	72	0078	6653
24	1114	8652	73	0071	6640
25	2.1048	2.8523	74	0065	6628
26	0987	8405	75	2.0058	2.6616
27	0932	8297	76	0052	6604
28	0881	8197	77	0046	6592
29	0834	8105	78	0040	6582
30	2.0790	2.8020	79	0035	6571
31	0750	7940	80	2.0029	2.6560
32	0711	7866	81	0023	6550
33	0676	7797	82	0018	6540
34	0642	7732	83	0012	6530
35	2.0611	2.7671	84	0007	6521
36	0581	7615	85	2.0003	2.6512
37	0553	7560	86	1.9998	6503
38	0527	7510	87	9994	6494
39	0502	7461	88	9989	6485
40	2.0478	2.7415	89	9985	6476
41	0456	7373	90	1.9980	2.6468
42	0435	7332	91	9976	6460
43	0414	7293	92	9972	6452
44	0395	7257	93	9968	6444
45	2.0377	2.7220	94	9964	6437
46	0359	7187	95	1.9960	2.6430
47	0342	7154	96	9956	6423
48	0326	7124	97	9952	6416
49	0310	7094	98	9949	6409
50	2.0296	2.7066	99	9945	6402
			100	1.9942	2.6396
			∞	1.9600	2.5758

From *Documenta Geigy Scientific Tables*, 7th ed., 1971, p. 44, by permission of the publishers Ciba-Geigy Ltd., Basel, Switzerland.

σ_p represents the standard error of the sampling distribution of repeated sample proportions p from samples of given size about $\mathcal{P}$.

Often these standard errors are replaced by sample estimates with the population standard errors estimated from $s/\sqrt{n}$ and

$\sqrt{p(1-p)/n}$, respectively. In this formulation, we are relying upon the similarity of the binomial distribution for repeatedly sampled proportions, when $\mathcal{P}$ is close to 50% and when the sample size is large, to the normal distribution of repeated sample means. This approximation is excellent when the sample size is large and p is close to 50%.

Example. HAS (Hospital Administration Services) uses a type of control chart in which, once a month, the performance of the hospital, as judged by any one of a number of indicators, is compared with the performance of other hospitals of comparable size.

In traditional control charts, the past performance of the plant (or hospital) is used to create standards against which current performance is judged. Typical questions that are answered by this approach are: "Is our current performance better or worse than our 'average' performance up to the present?" "Is our 'system' going out of control?" A sampling approach is used to answer these questions.

Example. A newly developed procedure enables the presence of hepatitis to be detected in blood drawn for transfusion. The test, however, is expensive and time-consuming.

The director of a blood bank arranged to have 1% of all blood for transfusion tested for the presence of hepatitis. Note that his object was not to screen out blood that might carry the hepatitis virus but rather to assure himself that the occurrence of such infected blood was kept at an acceptably low limit, since he had no control over the source of purchased blood.

After the first week, during which 3021 units of transfused blood were used, 30 units had been tested for hepatitis and only one contained the virus. The following Monday, a control chart was established, with the expectation of finding an infected unit as 1/30, or 3.3%. Assume that about 500 units were used each day and that we select 5 of these at random.

At this stage, we can proceed in a number of ways that are roughly equivalent. We can calculate the probability that, in a random sample of 5 tested units of blood, x units are infected.

Here x can take on any integer value from 0 to 5. Using the binomial distribution, we get

$$P(x \text{ infected out of } 5) = \binom{5}{x} (0.033)^x (1 - 0.033)^{5-x}$$

This is approximately equal to

$$\frac{5!}{x!\,(5-x)!} (0.033)^x$$

so that

$$
\begin{aligned}
P(1 \text{ infected}) &= \frac{5!}{1!\,4!} (0.033) \\
&= 5 \times 0.033 \\
&= 0.165,
\end{aligned}
$$

and

$$
\begin{aligned}
P(2 \text{ infected}) &= \frac{5!}{2!\,3!} (0.033)^2 \\
&= 10 \times 0.001089 \\
&= 0.01.
\end{aligned}
$$

These rough calculations tell us that if only 3.3% of all units of blood are infected, in a random sample of 5 the chance of finding 1 infected is about 17% and the chance of finding 2 infected is about 1%. The chance of finding 3, 4, or 5 infected is less than 1%. Therefore, the probability of finding 2 or more infected in a sample of 5 is less than 5%.

We can derive a rule of thumb from this calculation, namely, that if on a day on which two or more infected units are detected among the 5 units, the total consignment of blood is suspect and the proportion of infected blood is likely to be greater than the assumed 3% on which our calculations were based.

These conclusions are confirmed by tables showing exact 95% confidence limits for a proportion since, for a sample of size 5, an observed proportion of 20% (i.e., 1 in 5) can arise from populations with proportions between 5% and 85% with 95% confidence. In other words, our assumed proportion of 3.3% is "unacceptable" (i.e., an unlikely population proportion for two infected units to occur in a sample of 5). Thus, we have some evidence that the proportion of infected units has increased from our assumed frequency of 3.3%.

Another approach (and one which is frequently used in control charts) is to rely on the binomial approximation to the normal distribution. In this approach p is equated with the sample mean of a normal distribution, $\mathcal{P}$ is equated with the population mean of a normal distribution, and $\sqrt{\mathcal{P}(1 - \mathcal{P})/n}$ is equated with the standard error of the sample mean. The argument is that, just as for a normally distributed mean, 95% of all sample proportions should fall between

$$\mathcal{P} \pm 2 \sqrt{\frac{\mathcal{P}(1 - \mathcal{P})}{n}}$$

that is, between

$$0.033 \pm 2 \sqrt{\frac{0.033 \times 0.967}{5}}$$

or

$$0.033 \pm 2\sqrt{0.006382},$$
$$0.033 \pm 2 \times 0.080,$$
$$0.033 \pm 0.160,$$

that is, between 0 and 0.193. Now, forgetting that this is a two-tailed procedure in which we have lost one tail (since negative proportions are impossible), we note that the upper limit of these approximate 95% limits is 0.193 for sample proportions (in samples of size 5 from a population with 3.3% infected).

This means that 1 infected among 5, or 20%, is judged to be a "rare" event, since 20% lies outside the limits 0% to 19.3%. This result contradicts the above finding, because, if we used this procedure, we would reject the batch of blood if only 1 out of 5 units were found to be infected.

The example shows that the binomial approximation to the normal distribution is not to be trusted when the population proportion differs much from 50% *and* when the sample size is small. In this example, $\mathcal{P} = 3.3\%$, which is quite different from 50%. Also $n = 5$, which is quite small. (Generally samples of less than 50 are considered small.)

10.5 ACCEPTANCE SAMPLING

As the name **acceptance sampling** suggests, a (random) sample of a consignment is examined (by a buyer or consumer) and on the basis of this a decision is made whether to accept or reject the lot. The decision is made on the proportion of defective items found in the sample. Thus Table 7.2 can be used to test whether the sample comes from a population with an acceptable (population) proportion of defectives.

Example. A hospital contracts to buy 1000 disposable "sterile" anesthetic masks. It is agreed that no more than 0.5% of the masks should carry any pathogenic organisms. On delivery the hospital cultures the bacteria from a random sample of 25 of the masks and finds two of the masks to be potentially unsafe. Should the 1000 masks be returned? Clearly the masks should be rejected if more than 0.5% of them harbor pathogenic organisms. This is resolved by asking whether the 95% confidence interval for $p = 2/25$ contains 0.5%. Table 7.2 gives these limits as from 0.98% to 26.03%, which obviously excludes 0.5%. Therefore the lot should be rejected as potentially hazardous.

Acceptance sampling can also be applied to a continuous variable. Generally we ask whether the sample mean or standard deviation indicates that the population of items consigned to the buyer has an unacceptably high or low mean or standard deviation. These questions can, therefore, be couched in terms of confidence limits, and Tables 7.3 and 7.4 can be used to decide whether desired values of μ or σ lie within the 95% confidence limits for the observed sample statistic.

Example. A drug in tablet form is advertised as containing 30 mg of the active ingredient in each tablet. On getting his order from the manufacturer, a pharmacist performs five independent assays. The mean and standard deviation of these five assays are given as 35 ± 5 mg per tablet. Should the lot be rejected?
The 95% confidence limits for μ are from Table 7.3:

$$35 \pm 1.2416 \times 5 \equiv 28.792 \text{ to } 41.208 \text{ mg per tablet.}$$

On this basis, the lot should be accepted since the advertised potency for each tablet (30 mg) falls within these 95% confidence limits.

Acceptance sampling and control charts are thus seen as practical examples of decisions based on confidence limits and sampling distributions, respectively. The treatment given here is elementary (omitting, for example, a discussion of producer's risk). The reader is referred to other texts for specific details and tables.

EXERCISES

10.1   Explain the difference between Tables 7.3 and 10.4.

10.2   A decision whether or not to change from conventional bed sheets in the recovery room to disposable bed sheets must be made. The latter cost $0.25 each but are made to last for just 1 day (24 hours). The sheets now in use cost $5.00 a pair (in practice pairs of sheets are bought, since for each one in use, one will be at the laundry). The cost of laundering each pair of sheets is $1.50 each week. Hospital records show that these sheets have the following life times:

Number of weeks (midpoint of interval):	2	4	6	8	10	12	14	16
% Frequency	5	5	0	5	10	30	35	10

On the basis of these costs only, which is the better decision—to continue using laundered sheets or to begin replacing them with disposable bed sheets?

10.3   A hospital ship off the coast of Vietnam contains a surgical team. Usually, a helicopter full of critically wounded men arrives and the surgical team starts to treat the injured, one at a time. In order to optimize their effectiveness, the tea, first classifies the new arrivals and decides whom to treat according to an index of utility defined as follows:

$$\text{Utility} = \text{Probability of survival} \times 0.5$$
$$+ \text{ degree of normal function} \times 0.2$$
$$+ [1 - \text{age in years}/100] \times 0.1$$
$$+ \text{ status} \times 0.2$$

Status refers to whether the patient is either "friend or foe." "Friends" are given a status value of 1 and "foes" are given a status value of 0.2. (Note that each factor is defined between 0 and 1 and weighted to give a combined index of utility between 0 and 1, where 0 is low and 1 high). The party of injured is described as follows:

Patients no.	P(survival)	Normal function	Age	Status
1	0.25	0.95	25	Friend
2	0.80	0.20	55	Friend
3	0.50	0.50	5	Friend
4	0.05	0.80	20	Friend
5	0.66	0.75	30	Foe

In what order will the patients be treated?

10.4 The cost of sending a child through college is estimated to be $10,000. Therefore, a couple who have twins will have to pay $20,000 to put both their children through college simultaneously. For a premium of $2000, however, the couple can insure themselves so that if they have twins, the $20,000 will be paid by the insurance company. The probability of the woman's having twins is 0.15. Should the couple pay $2000 in premiums for this type of insurance?

10.5 The mean and standard deviation for the costs of drugs per patient-day for 50 patients hospitalized with respiratory tuberculosis is given as $2.30 ± $0.20. Calculate the 95% and 99% limits for the population of daily drug costs for all patients which this sample represents.

10.6 Nationally, 60% of 6-year-old children revealed on examination the eruption of the permanent first molars. A first-grade class of 30 children, in which the median age is 6 years, is examined orally. Using $(\overline{P} ± 2\sigma_p$, calculate the approximate 95% limits of the proportion of children in the class whose first molars have erupted.

LITERATURE CITED

Documenta Geigy Scientific Tables. 1962. 6th Ed. Ciba-Geigy Ltd., Basel, Switzerland.

Griffith, J. R. (Chairman). 1970. Report of the Task Force on Quantitative Methods. Association of University Programs in Hospital Administration, Washington, D.C.

Mainland, D. 1968. Notes on Biometry in Medical Research. Quality Control. Charts in Public Health, Note 19, pp. 19–24. V. A. Monograph 10-1, Suppl. 3. Veterans Administration, Washington, D.C.

Raiffa, H. 1968. Decision Analysis: Introductory Lectures on Choices under Uncertainty. Addison-Wesley Publishing Company Inc., Reading, Mass.

FURTHER READING

Barr, L. 1962. Optimum Purchasing Policy. Pub. No. 4, Operational Research Unit. p. 9. Oxford Regional Hospital Board, Oxford, England.

Benjamin, B. 1971. The Statistician and the Manager. J. Roy. Statist. Soc. Ser. A 134(1):1.

Fetter, R. B. 1967. The Quality Control System. Richard D. Irwin Inc., Homewood, Ill.

Jacquez, J. A. (Ed.) 1964. The Diagnostic Process. Malloy Lithographing, Ann Arbor, Michigan.

Sheldon, A., F. Baker and C. P. McLaughlin. 1970. Systems and Medical Care. MIT Press, Cambridge.

11
Forecasting Techniques

11.1 INTRODUCTION

The need for planning has increased with modern technology and the inertia of large organizations (Galbraith, 1972). This need is especially acute in the administration of health care systems, which in recent years has consumed a greater fraction of the national budget (8% in 1957). Forecasting techniques have naturally been developed in those areas in which prediction is most called for, e.g., the stock market, the national economy, military science. Consequently, different terms are used in different fields to describe the same technique or characteristic.

Forecasting combines techniques from regression analysis and the analysis of time series. In this chapter computational aspects are omitted, since most forecasters will tend to use one of a number of commonly available regression or forecasting computer programs. As elsewhere in this book, the emphasis is on understanding the meaning of the figures rather than on their calculation. A review of Section 2.2.3 ("Condensation of Information in Two Variables") and Section 2.2.4 ("Statistical Condensation for More than Two Variables") would be useful here for those readers not already familiar with the graphical presentation of data, e.g., the scattergram.

11.2 LINEAR REGRESSION BETWEEN TWO VARIABLES

The basic idea of regression is this: if y is our variable of interest and x is a known concomitant and if x and y have a high correlation (either positive or negative) then we construct an empirical relationship to tell us what value y will take as x changes.

Notice that we need to know the values that x takes for various values of y and we need to show that x and y are associated, otherwise there is little point in using regression techniques.

As an illustration, assume that we have, for a given year (say 1969), the number of hospital beds available and also the number of admissions to hospitals for each state in the United States in that year. The correlation coefficient for this data was 0.954 in 1969, so that $.954^2$ = 91% of the variation in one variable was associated with variation in the other. Now, in forecasting, we have the chicken and the egg problem. We have to decide which variable to use as the predictor for the other. In forecasting, this depends on the objective. It is conceivable that we may wish to use this information to check whether our state had either a high number of beds for a given number of admissions or had a high number of admissions for a given number of beds.

These are *different questions.* In the first, we predict the number of hospital beds required for a state with a given number of admissions. In the second, we predict the hospital utilization (number of admissions) for a given number of hospital beds. In each case, a different regression equation is used. It is conventional to call the predictor variable x and the predicted variable y. Generally, graphs show x plotted along the abscissa and y along the ordinate. Let us decide to call, for each state,

$$x = \text{number of hospital beds}$$

and

$$y = \text{number of admissions.}$$

Figure 11.1 shows the scattergram for this data. What is noticeable about the points? They appear to be scattered about the straight line drawn on the graph. This is the regression line of y on x. The

Figure 11.1. Number of hospital admissions (in thousands) by state against number of hospital beds (in thousands) in that state, 1969. (From *Hospital Statistics*, 44(2):501, August, 1970.)

criterion used to draw this line is to minimize the vertical deviations (squared) of the points from the line. A line that minimizes the sum of the horizontal deviations (squared) of the points from itself (i.e., the regression line of x on y) would not have the same slope.

The slope of the line y on x is called b, the **regression coefficient**. It measures the change in y for unit change in x. Thus, an increase of 1 bed will, it is predicted, be associated with an increase of between 16 and 17 in the number of admissions.

We write this regression line as

$$\hat{y} = 16.73x$$

where the hat on y reminds us that this is a value predicted from x and where 16.73 is the value of the regression coefficient. Different expressions for the calculation of the regression coefficient b may be given. The simplest, assuming we already know s_x and s_y, the standard deviation of x and y, and r the correlation of x and y, is

$$b_{y \cdot x} = r \frac{s_y}{s_x}$$

Note that the regression coefficient b has suffixes ($y \cdot x$) to represent 'y on x'. Often these suffixes are omitted if there is no ambiguity. It follows that b will be significantly different from zero if r is. A test of the significance of r, as in Section 9.7.1, is therefore also a test of the significance of b.

Note that in Figure 11.1, the graph cuts the y axis at 111,619. Thus in the regression equation, $\hat{y}$ is measured as the number of hospital admissions in excess of 111,619.

The equation of the regression line is now seen to be

$$\hat{y} - 111,619 = 16.73x$$

Rearranging, we get

$$\hat{y} = 111,619 + 16.73x$$

which is of the form of a straight line

$$\hat{y} = a + bx$$

where a is the intercept (i.e., the value of $\hat{y}$ when x is zero) and b the slope (i.e., the change in $\hat{y}$ for unit increase in x).

Let us assume that we know the age in years for each of the 89 men whose vital capacity is recorded in Table 5.2. Since vital capacity is affected by age and not the opposite, we set x = age and y = vital capacity. The correlation between x and y in this example is found to be -0.35. Since this is greater absolutely than the critical level of r for 5% significance (which, from Table 9.8 with n = 89 is 0.2084), we have demonstrated the existence of a significant association between x and y at the 5% level and we may proceed to calculate the linear regression equation. The mean and standard deviation of the 89 ages is 50.0 and 3.12 years and the mean and standard deviation of the 89 vital capacities is 4.80 and 0.89 liters respectively.

The regression coefficient b is then calculated as

$$b = \frac{-0.35 \times 0.89}{3.12} = -0.10$$

and the intercept a is calculated as (see Exercise 11.2 for the derivation)

$$a = \bar{y} - b\bar{x}$$
$$= 4.8 + 0.10 \times 50.00$$
$$= 9.8$$

The regression equation is then, where $\hat{y}$ is measured in liters and x in years,

$$\hat{y} = a + bx$$
$$= 9.8 - 0.10x$$

Thus, men aged 40 are predicted to have a vital capacity of 5.8 liters and men aged 60 a vital capacity of 3.8. Note that if we use this equation outside the age range 40 to 59, we get ridiculous results, e.g., at birth, baby boys have a vital capacity of 9.3 liters and as men approach 98 years of age, their vital capacity falls to zero!

Note also that this relationship does not necessarily describe the change in vital capacity in any given individual with age, e.g., an athlete in training would not necessarily show a fall in vital capacity. It is a common fallacy to apply relationships derived from aggregated units to individual units that make up that aggregate or to single units over time. For example, the relationship between average family income and the average number of years of higher education may be derived from aggregates of households in many census tracts. This relationship changes when we regress each household's income against years of higher education within a census tract. Likewise Susser (1973) quotes, as an example of this **aggregative fallacy,** the disparity between regional studies and studies of the individual on the relationship between hardness of drinking water and the risk of death from heart disease.

11.3 INTERPRETATION AND APPLICATION
OF SIMPLE LINEAR REGRESSION

The above section treats the fitting of regression as though the observations were known without error. In fact, the conventional calculation of a and b treats the problem as an example in statistical estimation. In other words, each observed y value is assumed to differ from its 'true' value. This deviation is represented by an error term in the model. The statistical interpretation of the estimated regression line then depends on assumptions about the 'error' term; namely, that the errors are independently distributed, that they follow a normal distribution, and that the standard deviation of these errors is constant as x increases. One can then estimate the standard errors of a and b, calculate their confidence limits, and test for the significance of differences between the observed estimates a and b and presumed population values α and β derived from other considerations. Often the computer program used to derive the regression equation will also provide these as additional options as well as calculating automatically the predicted value of y, $\hat{y}$ that corresponds to each x value and the difference, $\hat{y} - y$ between the predicted and observed values. These 'residuals', $\hat{y} - y$, can be further studied to check the appropriateness of the above assumptions concerning the error term in the regression model, and the appropriateness of the model itself, e.g., linearity.

A regression equation may be used for interpolation or extrapolation, i.e., for predicting the value of y expected if x took a value within the range observed or outside it. Of the two, interpolation is less hazardous, although bizarre situations exist in which interpolation can lead to a prediction far from the truth. The biggest danger is in using the regression equation for situations far removed from the original context. Thus, in the above example, we might use the regression equation to predict the number of annual hospital admissions for a new state entering the Union, given the number of hospital beds in that state. It would, however, be naive to apply this formula to, say, another country with a different system of health care (to say nothing about the possibility of different definition of terms, such as hospital bed or hospital admission).

The major difficulty in extrapolation is knowing how far one can trust the linear relationship. The straight line may be an adequate, though approximate, fit to a short section for which data exists and there is, therefore, little danger in departure from the linear model in interpolation. This is not true in extrapolating beyond the observed x values. In general, the farther away from the extreme x values the worse is the prediction. (For example, the number of admissions in a state with no hospital beds is 111,619!) It is, however, impossible to make a more precise statement without knowing the true relationship between y and x beyond the range of the observations. Each subject matter using forecasting emphasizes the necessity of an intimate knowledge of the system in order to judge how far one can safely extrapolate. In so doing, these specialists, whether in the stock market, the government or the Pentagon, are in fact incorporating additional subjective information (sometimes unconsciously) in making their judgments. This is called **sensitivity analysis** by some. Thus, in terms of the original example of hospital beds and admissions it would be unlikely if the same relationship held exactly in different years. In fact, the regression coefficients a and b change from

$$a = 111,619, \quad b = 16.73 \quad \text{in 1969}$$

to

$$a = 103,250, \quad b = 18.08 \quad \text{in 1970.}$$

Thus, a state with 10,000 beds would be predicted to have

$$\hat{y} = 111,619 + 16.73 \times 10,000 = 278,919$$

admissions using the 1969 regression equation and

$$\hat{y} = 103,250 + 18.08 \times 10,000 = 284,050$$

admissions using the 1970 regression equation.

11.4   TWO VARIABLES–
TRANSFORMATIONS AND CURVILINEAR REGRESSION

Often the original data is converted or transformed by the investigator or is taken from published tables in a transformed state. For example, a manpower study might seek to relate the number of orthodontists per 100,000 population to the number of persons under 21 per 100,000 population. Here the conversion to rates per 100,000 is redundant. Multiplying or dividing by or adding or subtracting a constant to each observation will not change the correlation coefficient between the two original variables, although the regression equation will change because of the change of the scale. Most conversions of the underlying units will not, therefore, affect the strength of the association between the variables, e.g., conversion of temperature from Centigrade to Fahrenheit.

Known relationships that are curvilinear can be converted to a straight line relationship by an appropriate transformation of one or other variables. Thus, it can be shown (Froggatt et al., 1969) that frequencies of visits to the doctor follow the negative binomial distribution. Knowing the distribution suggests that linearizing relation, which is

$$y = x \, f_x / f_{x-1} \text{ plotted against } x$$

where x is the annual number of visits to the doctor and f_x is the frequency of the population with this number of visits.

The above was a specific example. In general, four types of transformations are commonly used to linearize a relationship. These transformations involve plotting the reciprocal, square root, logarithm, or probit of the original observation. In the following we give some examples of these four transformations.

Examples.

Reciprocal Transformations

The Michaelis-Menton formula relates the velocity V of an enzyme reaction to the concentration S of the substrate by

$$V = \frac{V_{\max} \cdot S}{\text{Constant} + S}$$

where $V_{\max}$ = maximum velocity at high substrate concentrations.

To linearize this relationship, we plot the reciprocals $1/V$ against $1/S$ for then

$$1/V = 1/V_{\max} + \text{constant} \cdot 1/S$$

which is the form of a straight line. The intercept $1/V_{\max}$ and the constant slope may then be estimated from the regression of $1/V$ against $1/S$.

Square Root Transformations

The location of health care facilities affects their use. Increasing the number of such facilities will decrease the average distance travelled according to the relationship (Donabedian, 1973).

Reduction in average distance travelled =
(Increase in the number of health care facilities)$^{-\frac{1}{2}}$

A straight line relationship should, therefore, result from a graph of y, reduction in average distance travelled, against $1/\sqrt{x}$, where x is the increase in the number of health care facilities.

Logarithmic Transformations

The above examples are cases in which the transformation that linearized the relationship involved changing the power of one variable. When the functional relationship is multiplicative or when the power of the variable is unknown, taking logarithms will often yield a straight line. Thus, surface area in square centimeters (S) is related approximately to body height, H (in centimeters) and body weight W in kg by the relationship

$$S = 71.84 \, H^{0.725} \, W^{0.425}$$

Taking logarithms of both sides of this equation yields

$$\log S = 1.8564 + 0.725 \log H + 0.425 \log W$$

giving straight line relationships between surface area and height for constant weight or surface area and weight for constant height when transformed into logarithms. (Logarithms to the base 10 are used.)

The hyperbolic equation

$$y = c/x^d$$

has been proposed for the relationship between frequency of visits to the doctor (y) and distance travelled (x). Here c and d are constants fitted from the data, which vary from urban to rural counties (Donabedian, 1973). The values of c and d may be estimated from a graph using semi-log paper or by transforming to logarithms.

Jelinek (1967) likewise uses a logarithmic transformation in relating the number of hours of direct patient care per patient day with the available number of nurses. He relates the logarithm of the amount of non-productive time per patient day to the size of the available staff. In the first case, therefore, he linearizes his relationship by taking logarithms of x, the independent or predictor variable, whereas in the second application he takes logarithms of y, the dependent or predicted variable, to effect a straight line relationship.

Probit Transformations

Finally, among these examples, is the probit transformation of drug response often regressed against log dose (the dosage). The cumulative percentage of patients who have responded to an increasing dose or dosage of a drug gives a characteristic sigmoid curve when plotted against dose or dosage. The probit transformation in effect transforms this cumulative response into the equivalent number of standard deviations from the average (which is arbitrarily labeled 5). Since ± 2 standard deviations exclude approximately 2.5% in each tail of a normal frequency distribution this means that a 2.5% response becomes a probit of $(5 - 2) = 3$ and that a 97.5% response will correspond to a probit of $(5 + 2) = 7$. In short, the cumulative percent responding is converted into its equivalent normal deviate plus 5.

The linearizing effect of each of these four transformations can be seen graphically, but how to discriminate between two alternative transformations? Assume we have three different models (y on x; y on $\sqrt{x}$; y on log x) then we could calculate the correlation coefficient for each pair and compare these or their squares to find which model gives the best linear 'fit.' It is probably unnecessary to apply a significance test in the comparison of these correlations. Either we get a high correlation with one of these or we do not. If not, it is possible that either another transformation should be tried or that no model can be found that will significantly relate one variable to the other.

In this section relationships have been considered as though they were exact. In fact, each model fitted to real data will generate a residual error that is the difference between the observed and fitted value of y for that value of x. Usually, statisticians apply transformations, not to linearize a relationship, but to produce independent residuals or to generate equal variability around the fitted relationship. Linearizing or simplifying transformations may, therefore, have the opposite effect of producing non-independent errors or an error term that varies with the level of x. It is always good practice, therefore, to examine the residuals remaining after a regression model has been fitted. In Section 11.10, we give several procedures for testing these residuals for randomness or independence.

11.5 MORE THAN TWO VARIABLES—MULTIPLE REGRESSION

11.5.1 Number of Variables Fixed

We often can improve our ability to forecast by introducing additional correlated variables. Thus, body weight for males is related to both height and age. Unfortunately, it is difficult to graph a relationship among three variables and impossible to graph a relationship among more than three variables. Another complication is that the relationship derived by adding another predictor variable is not the sum of the two simple relationships. Thus, the regression of weight on height and age cannot be calculated by adding the expressions relating weight to height and weight to age. The two predictor variables, age and height, are themselves related. To estimate the best fitting regression, one would use a least-squares procedure (each computer center has a number of different programs for doing these regression calculations). To ascertain whether the addition of age as a predictor variable was advantageous, one would evaluate the percentage of total variation "explained" by the model in each case and compare these as shown in the numerical example that follows.

Similarly, in order to test whether a given transformation increased in the fit, one would use the same approach. Thus, rather than fitting

$$\text{Weight} = a + b\ \text{Age} + c\ \text{Height}$$

one might try fitting

$$\text{Weight} = a + b\ \text{Age} + c\ \log \text{Height}$$

In both of these a, b, c, are regression constants to be estimated by least squares. (They will take different values in the different models.) Then, as before, we could compare percentage of total variation explained by each. This is done by calculating and comparing the multiple regression coefficient or its square in each case. The multiple regression coefficient squared is simply the ratio of the sum of squares of deviations of the predicted values about the mean to the total sum of squares of deviations of the original observations about the mean.

The transformation may apply also to the predicted variable. Thus in relating y, the size of the community served by a group of hospitals, to x, the population density, and to z, the number of hospital beds per 1000 persons, the regression model fitted was (Commission on Hospital Care, 1957)

$$\log y = a + b \log x + c \log z$$

Another example of a transformed dependent variable is given by Peacock et al. (in press). In this study, multiple regression was used to investigate the effect of housing on reported morbidity. The basic observation was the number of episodes of illness reported in a given period by those of a given age and sex living in a specified type of housing. The preliminary dependent variable was, therefore, the episode rate; i.e., the number of episodes of illness divided by the number of persons at risk in that period, housing type, age, and sex group. Because of the different age/sex composition of those living in different housing types, it was necessary to allow for these age/sex variations. This was not done, however, by including age and sex as predictor variables in the regression (this would have made the regression unwieldy) but by directly standardizing the episode rates for age and sex (Fleiss, 1973). This gave a directly standardized episode rate for each of eight housing types in each of four periods. Since there was little direct interest in the period effect per se, this information was used in calculating the error term. The final model, therefore, was reduced to

$$\text{D.S.R.}_{ij} = \overline{\text{D.S.R.}} + h_i + e_{ij}$$

where

D.S.R.$_{ij}$ = episode rate of the ith housing type in the jth period standardized directly for age and sex
$\overline{D.S.R.}$ = the mean of these 32 standardized rates

and

h_i = effect of housing type i on $\overline{D.S.R}$

and

e_{ij} = an error term for the ith housing type in the jth period.

Thus, an investigation that started out conceptually as a complex multiple regression was reduced to a simple one-factor analysis of variance.

This example illustrates the well-known fact that the analysis of variance is just a special case of regression analysis. Classically, regression is based on continuous predictor variables, whereas the analysis of variance is based on a multiple classification of several discrete factors at several different levels. However, with appropriate coding the two procedures are equivalent and may be calculated using the same general linear model computer program. (Note that computer programs for regression are classified as appropriate for models that are either linear or non-linear *in terms of the regression coefficients.* Thus:

$$\hat{y} = a + bx + cx^2$$

is a linear model in a, b, and c whereas

$$\hat{y} = ax^b$$

is a non-linear model in a and b.)

11.5.2 Variable Number of Variables

More often than not, it is unknown which variables should be included in a multiple regression equation or which model should be used. Empirically, the linear model is used as a first approximation when the true relationship is unknown. Repeated multiple regressions are calculated to find the sub-set of all potential variables that maximizes the multiple regression coefficient for a given fixed number of variables. Many regression programs include step-wise procedures by which the optimal number of variables may be empirically determined.

A particular type of multiple regression is one in which the relationship between two variables y and x is curvilinear but unknown as to its form. In this case, powers of x may be introduced to allow for this non-linear component. Thus, it is known that the number of people seen weekly by doctors in private practice falls off with the age of the physician (Donabedian, 1973) in a curvilinear manner. One can, therefore, form a multiple regression equation from two variables by using powers of x, i.e., the **polynomial**

$$y = a + bx + cx^2 + dx^3 + \text{etc.}$$

This model is computationally identical to the general multiple regression equation

$$y = a + bx + cz + dw + \text{etc.}$$

especially if these predictor variables (x, z, w) are themselves related.

Brooks and Beenhakker (1964) demonstrate the use of an exploratory multiple regression approach in attempting to predict the number of beds needed by a hospital to meet future demands. They separately determine a different regression for each of 17 specialities. These are based on different sub-sets of 117 factors. Initially, they determined the correlation between the number of beds needed in each of the 17 specialities and each of these 117 factors (i.e., $17 \times 117 = 1989$ correlations!) in order to select predictor variables for each regression equation. The form in which each variable entered the regression equation was then determined by graphing each against each selected predictor variable and comparing the resultant correlations. (All of this could have been done on the computer.) Finally, they constructed their regression equations by a forward selection procedure in which that variable that best predicts y is first entered into the regression. The next step is to calculate that variable that, when added

Table 11.1. The amount of variation explained (R^2) and the coefficients of different regression models fitted to 1969 and 1970 data on admissions (y) and hospital beds (x) in 51 states

	1969				
	R^2	a	b	c	d
Linear $\hat{y} = a + bx$	91%	111,619	16.73	–	–
Quadratic $\hat{y} = a + bx + cx^2$	95%	–10,008	25.22	–.00006	–
Cubic $\hat{y} = a + bx + cx^2 + dx^3$	96%	62,378	16.80	.0001	0
	1970				
	R^2	a	b	c	d
Linear $\hat{y} = a + bx$	92%	103,250	18.08	–	–
Quadratic $\hat{y} = a + bx + cx^2$	95%	–12,704	26.47	–.00006	–
Cubic $\hat{y} = a + bx + cx^2 + dx^3$	96%	65,775	17.05	.0001	0

Source: *Hospitals* (1970) 44(2):501 and *Hospitals* (1971) 45(2):490.

to this first variable, maximizes R^2, the percentage of the variation accounted for by regression on two variables, etc. This procedure would finally exhaust the variables potentially available for prediction. In practice, however, inclusion of new variables stops whenever the increases in R^2 falls below some reasonable percentage specified by the investigator.

Returning to the original example of regression of hospital admission on beds, Table 11.1 shows the effect of fitting quadratic and cubic terms (i.e., terms to represent the square of the number of beds and the cube of the number of beds). Fitting a linear regression to 1969 date accounts for 91% of the state-to-state variation in admissions. Fitting an additional quadratic term explains an additional 4% of the total variation whereas the cubic term adds only a further 1%. The table shows that d, the coefficient of the cubic term, is effectively zero (the computer printed out a decimal point and eight zeros). The cubic polynomial

$$\hat{y} = a + bx + cx^2 + dx^3$$

is therefore unnecessarily complicated. Dropping off the last term (as the one which contributes least to the R^2 value) we have yet to decide whether to use a linear or quadratic regression.

In other words, is it sufficient to use a linear regression

$$\hat{y} = a + bx$$

or is it better to use an additional term in x^2, which implies that

$$\hat{y} = a + bx + cx^2?$$

It should be noted that adding terms to a regression model always increases the percentage of variation explained by the analysis. Thus, in Table 11.1 adding a term in x^3 is seen to increase R^2 in that model by 1%, even though the regression coefficient of x^3 is smaller than 10^{-8}. We must, therefore, seek a regression equation that gives us the largest R^2 value with the smallest number of terms. One rule of thumb might be to include additional terms only when the increase in R^2 is more than half of the previous R^2 value. Thus, if R^2 = 50% with two terms a and b (linear regression), a quadratic term would be introduced only if $R^2 > 75%$ with three terms (a, b, and c), and a cubic if $R^2 > 88%$ with four terms (a, b, c, and d), etc. By this rule, we would be restricted to a linear model in Table 11.1, since R^2 = 91% with two terms in 1969.

We could also do a test of significance on the increase in R^2 by the introduction of an additional regression term. Assume that your computer program gives a value for R^2 for each regression equation fitted. Then, for a given set of n observations you may have fitted a regression model with $(p - 1)$ regression coefficients and got the appropriate R^2 value. Call this R^2_{p-1}. To test whether or not the addition of one more term to this model is justified you would calculate R^2_p, the appropriate R^2 value for the model with p terms. The test statistic is then, following Kempthorne (1952)

$$\frac{(R_p^2 - R_{p-1}^2)(n - p)}{(1 - R_p^2)}$$

This is calculated and compared against F with $n' = 2$ and $n'' = n - p$ + 1 in Table 9.7a. If, for example, the test statistic is larger than the critical value of F given in Table 9.7, then the additional term is judged to be a significant improvement in R^2 (at the 5% level).

We are now in a position to compare the need for quadratic term in Table 11.1. The test statistic for 1969 data is

$$\frac{(.95 - .91) \cdot (51 - 3)}{(1 - .95)} = 38.4$$

This is compared against an F value in Table 9.7a with $n' = 2$ and $n'' = 51 - 3 + 1 = 49$. This value is about 4, so the test statistic is much greater than the critical value, implying that a quadratic term does add a significant amount to the predictability of the regression. Note that our earlier rule of thumb (which was to incorporate the quadratic term if $R_3^2/R_2^2 > 1.5$) resulted in the conclusion that a linear model was sufficient. (This is not unexpected, since different criteria are expected to lead to different conclusions. Do not be afraid to use your own rule of thumb; this is an area in which there is no strictly rigorous statistical procedure.)

Table 11.1 also shows the same results for 1970 data. Note that while R^2 for a given model is the same (within 1%) for 1969 and 1970 data, the regression coefficients differ somewhat. However, the values of a, b, c are more alike for the same regression model in different years than are these coefficients in the same year for different models.

A regression equation can be used either to extrapolate or to examine how deviant an observed value is from the regression curve (which in some sense represents the average relationship between x and y). Table 11.2 compares the number of admissions in Virginia in 1969 and 1970 with the number predicted by the 1969 and 1970 linear and quadratic regressions. It can be seen, for its number of hospital beds, that Virginia has 16% and 19% higher admissions than would be expected from a linear regression in

Table 11.2. Comparison of actual admissions in Virginia with predictions based on linear and quadratic regression derived from all 50 states in 1969 and 1970

| | Actual values | | Predicted value/actual value | | | |
| | | | Linear regression | | Quadratic regression | |
Year	Beds	Admissions	1969	1970	1969	1970
1969	35,181	604,667	1.16	1.22	1.33	1.40
1970	35,175	622,199	1.13	1.19	1.29	1.36

1969 and 1970, respectively. Using a quadratic model, this excess becomes 33% and 36%, respectively, in the years 1969 and 1970. If now we attempt to predict Virginia's admissions from the number of hospital beds in that year, but using a regression equation calculated from the hospital data of the adjacent year, we find that we can predict 1970 admissions from the 1969 regression better than we predict the 1969 linear regressions. Thus, we are 13% high in predicting 1970 admission from the 1969 linear regression as compared to 22% high in predicting 1969 from 1970 regressions.

This table illustrates the need for confidence limits on regression equations so that we can describe the scatter of the observations about the fitted line or curve. It also illustrates the need for standard errors of the regression coefficients and for sensitivity analysis of the forecasting ability of the regression in time and space. Such topics are beyond the scope of this expository treatment. It is suggested that, if interested in pursuing these ideas, the reader consult some of the references listed in "Further Reading" at the end of this chapter.

11.6 TIME SERIES OVERVIEW

In the preceding sections of this chapter, regression techniques have been developed for a sample of observations (y, x) or (y, x, z, etc.) in which each observation is an independent realization of the underlying relationship occurring at a given point in time. Now we turn our attention to a sequential series of observations, occurring at time points represented by the suffix t. Thus, a patient's temperature chart is a simple example of a **time series**, as is a daily hospital census. Here, we restrict ourselves to simple time series in which only one time-dependent observation is recorded. Multiple time series in which one variable (say the Gross National Product) is related to a number of other variables, all recorded sequentially in time, are not covered.

Time series are analyzed with two very different objectives, either to forecast the future or to investigate the underlying causes of the variation. Thus, a hospital administrator is more interested in forecasting future bed needs than in studying the origins of this need. On the other hand, a research neurologist is more interested in understanding the biological causes for the electrical rhythms of the brain than in predicting the next EEG value. Fortunately, both objectives are broadly achieved by a common set of analytical procedures that have been developed for time series. Since many of these procedures are complex, both the forecaster and the researcher will tend to depend on computer programs for actual computations. A review of these techniques is essential for intelligent use of such programs. As ever, the user must bring to the problem his own perception and knowledge of the system.

In many sets of historical data, the interval between observations is fixed by the recording system, e.g., a daily bed census. In others, such as the monitoring of continuous biological systems, the sampling fraction, i.e., the number of observations per cycle, is set by the observer. The best sampling fraction depends on one's interest. For example, if one were not interested in seasonal variation, then one observation per annum would be sufficient. On the other hand, if seasonality were of primary importance, then observations should be taken quarterly or even at monthly intervals. In biological applications, from five to ten equally spaced observations should be taken per cycle to insure the recovery of the input signal. In the remainder of this chapter we shall assume that observations occur at equally spaced time intervals.

The standard approach to analyzing a time series is to assume that it is best described by one or more components plus a random error. The non-random components that are detected and estimated are a **trend**, a **cycle**, and a **seasonal effect**. For each, we fit a term to represent that component and then examine the residual time series (the differences between the observed time series and the one predicted by the model) for other components. Note that residuals are only identical to the error term when the perfect model has been fitted exactly. Residuals therefore are composed of the error term, other components not yet fitted, and also deviations introduced by the estimation procedure. In practice, any fitting procedure will distort the residuals.

Before we begin this decomposition of a time series into its components we may adjust the data to make allowance for different periods, e.g., by converting all calendar dates to a 30-day month, by converting to constant dollars to remove inflation, and by aggregating days into weeks to remove weekend effects.

11.7   TRENDS AND MOVING AVERAGES

The essence of a pure trend (one without an error term) is that it is smooth. As such it should be well represented, at least locally, by a polynomial based on time as the independent variable. Thus, a linear trend can be represented as:

$$y_t = a + bt$$

where a and b are unknown constants.

Since it follows that

$$y_{t+1} = a + b(t + 1), \text{ etc.}$$

the average of y_t, y_{t+1}, y_{t+2} is:

$$\frac{y_t + y_{t+1} + y_{t+2}}{3} = \frac{a + bt + a + b(t + 1) + a + b(t + 2)}{3}$$

$$= a + b(t + 1) = y_{t+1}.$$

Thus, an average of an odd number of successive observations in a linear trend is equal to the middle value of the set averaged. This averaging is therefore able to uncover a trend in the presence of random error, since, to a large extent, in the averaging procedure the random errors in successive observations will cancel. The term **moving average** is used to describe this procedure, since, in each successive calculation, the first observation in the last average is omitted and a new observation is added at the end of the list of numbers to be averaged.

Curvilinear trends can be similarly detected and removed. To do so, one weights successive values according to the values given by the degree of the polynomial fitted. Kendall (1973) gives these weights for calculating moving averages to remove different types of trend. Weights for end effects and for forecasting one term ahead of the series are likewise given. Such tables may of course be redundant if a computer program is used. Unfortunately, the removal of a trend will also tend to smooth the residuals, resulting in a positive serial correlation between successive residuals. A subsequent test of randomness on these residuals may therefore detect the spurious serial correlation, with the implication that the series originally contained a seasonal effect when this is not so. Likewise, true seasonal effects may be affected by the removal of a trend by moving averages. Thus, a long oscillation will to some extent be treated as part of the trend and will tend to be removed by the moving average.

11.8 EXPONENTIAL SMOOTHING

Exponential smoothing is a type of averaging in which less weight is given to the older observations. The prediction of the next observation is the weighted average of the last observation and its predicted value. Thus, successive predictions are related by the recursive equation

$$\hat{y}_{t+1} = \gamma \cdot y_t + (1 - \gamma) \cdot \hat{y}_t$$

where $\hat{y}_t$ is the exponentially smoothed prediction for the time period t and γ is the weighting factor. For $\gamma = 0.1$, the last observation will have a weight of 10%, the next to last 9%, the next 8.1%, the next 7.3%, etc. In exponential smoothing, the weights fall off geometrically, e.g., the weight is $\gamma(1 - \gamma)^n$ for the nth observation before the current one. The effect of changing γ can be investigated empirically in past time series to see if this improves the prediction. Generally, a low γ is used for the smoother time series and a high γ for one that is rapidly fluctuating. Values of γ above .3 are rarely used, because then the series is fluctuating so rapidly that prediction is worthless. The results of exercise 11.8 at the end of this chapter have been used to illustrate the relative ability of a moving average and exponential smoothing to track an observed time series (Figure 11.2) and exercises 11.9 and 11.10 to demonstrate the effect of changing γ from .3 to .1 (Figure 11.3).

Exponential smoothing is appropriate to predict or to track a long series that is composed of a constant term plus random variation. Exponential smoothing may also be applied to predict the next value in a time series with a definite trend. Here, we regard the predicted values as a time series in their own right

$$\cdots\cdots\hat{y}_{t-2}, \hat{y}_{t-1}, \hat{y}_t, \hat{y}_{t+1}\cdots\cdots$$

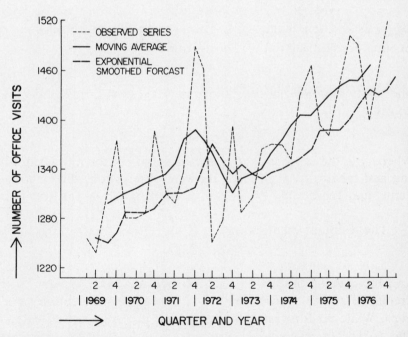

Figure 11.2. Results of exercise 11.8 comparing the ability of a moving average and exponential smoothing to track an observed time series (Table 11.4).

Figure 11.3. Effect of changing γ from 0.3 to 0.1 in forecasts of the number of births expected in the next 12 hours (Exercises 11.9, 11.10).

and apply exponential smoothing to this series of predicted values to get

$$\hat{\hat{y}}_{t+1} = \gamma\hat{y}_t + (1 - \gamma)\hat{\hat{y}}_t$$

where γ is the same weighting factor as used in the initial smoothing and where y_t, $\hat{y}_t$, $\hat{\hat{y}}_t$ are the raw observation, the smoothed value, and the doubly smoothed value, respectively, at time point t.

The resultant prediction is

$$\hat{\hat{y}}_t = \hat{y}_t + (\hat{y}_t - \hat{\hat{y}}_t),$$

i.e., the original prediction plus a correction term to allow for the trend. Of course, in the absence of a trend this correction term is zero. While no forecast will ever predict a change not reflected in the past data, the above system will at least track reasonably faithfully a random time series in which systematic trends appear and disappear.

11.9 PERIODICITY

Under this heading, we consider both seasonal effects and naturally occurring cycles. The presence of cycles may easily be detected by inspection or by **spectral analysis** (for a description of spectral analysis, see Brown [1963]). Examples of time series with cyclic components abound in medicine and physiology because of the circadian rhythms of the body, for example, body temperature and the pump-like actions of the heart and lungs, both normal and abnormal, e.g., Cheyne-Stoke breathing and auricular fibrillation. Seasonal effects are also well recognized in health care, e.g., the daily cycle of the number of births in an obstetrical facility, the peak of emergency admissions at the weekend in urban hospitals, the average monthly census, demand curves and inventory depletions, and the incidence of infectious disease. Seasonal effects may be recognized visually as peaks or troughs that occur at the same period each year. It is also helpful in defining the existence of a seasonal component to know its causation, e.g., that the death rate among the elderly is higher in the winter because of the weather.

One approach to the smoothing or prediction of periodic effects that appears to be tied to specific time periods is to consider each interval in the period separately. Thus, one could extract only the temperature recorded at 8 A.M. in successive days or only the bed census for April in successive years. Such a time series would then be considered as one without a seasonal component and so one could apply moving averages or exponential smoothing to the sub-sample of observations. Two other approaches to estimating or removing a seasonal component are to decompose the time series using moving averages or to estimate the components using regression analysis. How a moving average will remove a trend to reveal the seasonal component is illustrated here by using fictitious data to represent average bed costs over the past 70 years. Table 11.3 shows how we construct a hypothetical time series (column c) by adding a quadratic term x^2 (column a) to a periodic term (± 5) (column b). We almost recover this periodic term as the residual (column e) after a moving average (column d) is subtracted from the time series (column c). The moving average used was

$$(y_{t-1} + 2y_t + y_{t+1})/4$$

Table 11.3. Hypothetical hospital costs per bed per day showing how a simple moving average can remove a quadratic trend to reveal a periodicity

	Quadratic component (a)	Quinquennial variation (b)	Time series (c = a + b)	Moving average (d)	Residual (e = c − d)
1910–14	9	+5	14	–	–
1915–19	16	–5	11	16.50	–5.50
1920–24	25	+5	30	25.50	4.50
1925–29	36	–5	31	36.50	–5.50
1930–34	49	+5	54	49.50	4.50
1935–39	64	–5	59	64.50	–5.50
1940–44	81	+5	86	81.50	4.50
1945–49	100	–5	95	100.50	–5.50
1950–54	121	+5	126	121.50	4.50
1955–64	144	–5	139	144.50	–5.50
1960–69	169	+5	174	169.50	4.50
1965–69	196	–5	191	196.50	–5.50
1970–74	225	+5	230	225.50	4.50
1975–79	256	–5	251	–	–

giving, for the first entry in column d,

$$(14 + 2 \times 11 + 30)/4 = 16.50$$

To illustrate the regression approach let us assume that we know each day's bed costs. We then can aggregate to find each month's average bed costs per day over the 70-year period (1910–1980). Further, let us assume that the periodic component shows an annual cycle. We then consider the 70 values for each month as a separate time series.

Let y_{ij} equal the average bed costs per day for the ith month of the jth year. Then y_{ij} will be considered as the dependent variable in 12 separate regressions, one for each month. To derive the "independent" variable in the regression we consider the whole time series y_{ij}, $i = 1$ to 12, $j = 1910$ to 1980, and calculate for each month the centered trend value x_{ij} based on the surrounding 13 months. Thus, the trend value for April 1974 would be:

$$x_{4,74} = [y_{10,73} + 2y_{11,73} + 2y_{12,73} + 2y_{1,74} + 2y_{2,74} + 2y_{3,74} + 2y_{4,74} + 2y_{5,74} + 2y_{6,74} + 2y_{7,74} + 2y_{8,74} + 2y_{9,74} + y_{10,74}] \div 24$$

We now have for the month of April, 70 pairs of observations $(y_{4,j}, x_{4,j})$, $j = 1910 - 1980$, and we can estimate the regression coefficients for April in the linear regression equation

$$y_{4,j} = a_4 + b_4 x_{4j} + e_{4j}$$

Having estimated all 12 pairs of regression coefficients a_i, b_i, we average these to get the smoothed bed cost as

$$\hat{y}_{ij} = \bar{a} + \bar{b} x_{ij} \text{ where } \bar{a} = \sum_{1}^{12} a_i/12 \text{ and } \bar{b} = \sum_{1}^{12} b_i/12$$

To remove the seasonal component from monthly bed costs, we would calculate

$$\hat{y}_{ij} \text{ (adjusted)} = \frac{\hat{y}_{ij} - (a_i - \bar{a})}{(b_i - \bar{b})}$$

Plotting these seasonally adjusted values should reveal a trend if it exists.

The above regression method, however, is rather cumbersome in that it estimates 24 parameters, requiring a considerable computational effort on a considerable body of data. In addition, the method assumes that the travel and seasonal effects have remained reasonably constant with time. In practice, therefore, the regression approach to seasonality requires a long stable series with invariant components. These are rare.

11.10   TESTS OF RESIDUALS

Estimation and removal of a systematic component from a time series requires a test of the randomness of the resultant residuals. If the test fails, this means that the decomposition has not yet been completed. The test of randomness is, however, to some extent subjective, since the test chosen will depend on whether one is testing against trend, cycle, or seasonal effect. Consider as an example of a time series the average monthly census of a hospital. We first consider whether or not these observations can be described as fully random. A random time series is one in which the graph of the data would not be greatly altered in appearance if the order in which observations were plotted were altered.

We define a **turning point** as a local peak or trough, i.e., an observation that is higher or lower than either of the observations before and after it. Then, in a random series the number of turning points is approximately normally distributed with mean $2(n - 2)/3$ and variance $(16n - 29)/90$, where n is the number of observations in the series (counting successive observations that are identical as one point). We can, therefore, compare the number of turning points against its expectation from a random series using a t test (see Section 9.4.2). This test should indicate cycles or seasonal effects in the time series but may not detect a mild trend in the presence of marked random fluctuation. A better test of a presumed random series to detect the existence of a trend is to count the number of observations in the series that are larger than their immediate predecessor. This number is likewise approximately normally distributed, with mean $(n - 1)/2$ and variance $(n + 1)/12$.

11.11   FORECASTING FORMULAS

Suppose we wish to forecast a time series y_t that we suspect to contain a trend and a seasonal component. We then have to estimate the trend and seasonal effects at each point in time, remove them and predict the resultant smoothed series forward. To do this, we need to recursively estimate four formulas. For monthly data with a 12-month cycle, the forecast for next month y_{t+1} will be the estimated trend R_t at time t added to the smoothed value of the series D_t at time t, all multiplied by an inflation factor S_{t-12+1} to allow for the anticipated seasonal change from time t to time $t+1$.

In symbols this is (following Phillip [1970]):

$$\hat{y}_{t+1} = (D_t + R_t) \cdot S_{t-12+1}$$

where

> D_t represents the "deseasonalized," or smoothed, value of the series at time t,
>
> R_t represents the trend in a unit interval $(t-1, t)$,
>
> and S_t represents the seasonal factor for the month and year represented by time t. (To forecast n months ahead, one replaces S_{t-12+1} with S_{t-12+n}.)

To calculate D_t, R_t and S_t recursively, we need to specify the value of the exponential smoothing constant γ (generally, between 0.1 and 0.3). The recursive formulas for calculating these three values are of the exponential smoothing form

$$\hat{X}_t = \gamma X_t + (1 - \gamma)\hat{X}_{t-1}$$

where here X represents any one of the three variables calculated.

To get the smoothed or deseasonalized value D_t we combine a current estimate with a predicted value. Since we know D_{t-1}, the value of the smoothed series at time $t-1$, and since we also have a trend value R_{t-1} for that point in time, we add these to get $(D_{t-1} + R_{t-1})$ as our predicted value of D_t. The current estimate of D_t is obtained by dividing y_t by the seasonal factor for that period. Since this is unknown we are forced to use our last estimate S_{t-12} for monthly data or S_{t-4} for quarterly data. The exponentially smoothed value of D_t, the deseasonalized series, is then:

$$D_t = \gamma(y_t/S_{t-12}) + (1 - \gamma)(D_{t-1} + R_{t-1})$$

S_t, the seasonal factor at time t is likewise estimated as a weighted combination of the same seasonal factor in the last cycle $(S_{t-12}$ if monthly, S_{t-4} if quarterly) and a current value. The current seasonal value is obtained by dividing the current observation y_t by the estimated smoothed or deseasonalized value D_t. The expression is then:

$$S_t = \gamma \, (y_t/D_t) + (1 - \gamma)S_{t-12}$$

Thus, R_t, the trend value at time t is a weighted average of R_{t-1}, the trend at $t - 1$, and the current trend estimated as the difference between D_t and D_{t-1}. In symbols this is:

$$R_t = \gamma(D_t - D_{t-1}) + (1 - \gamma)R_{t-1}$$

Finally, to start these calculations, assume $D_1 = y_1$, $S_1 = 1$, $R_1 = 0$ and that all prior values of S also equal one.

Example. We illustrate this procedure numerically using quarterly data, since the calculations are less cumbersome for quarterly than monthly data. To adapt the above formulas to quarterly data, replace S_{t-12} by S_{t-4}.

Table 11.4 gives, in the column headed y_t, the number of persons seen quarterly by a dentist in the last eight years. It is clear that the numbers exhibit a mild trend (from 1254 to 1520 visits per quarter) over the eight-year period. The mean number of visits in each of the four quarters is 1355, 1310, 1364, and 1436, respectively, so that there is some indication of a seasonal effect also.

Here we illustrate the initial expressions to start the recursive calculations.

1969 The initial values are specified as

$$D_1 = y_1 = 1254$$
$$S_1 = 1$$
$$R_1 = 0$$
$$\hat{y}_2 = y_1 = 1254$$

Therefore, the calculations proper start for the second quarter, for which $y_2 = 1234$. We take $\gamma = .2$ throughout.

$$D_2 \quad = .2(y_2/S_{2-4}) + .8(D_1 + R_1)$$
$$= .2 \times 1234/1 + .8 \times 1254$$

$$= 1250.0$$

$$S_2 \quad = .2(y_2/D_2) + .8\, S_{2-4}$$

$$= .2 \times 1234/1250.0 + .8 \times 1$$

$$= 0.9974$$

$$R_2 \quad = .2(D_2 - D_1) + .8\, R_1$$

$$= .2 \times (1250 - 1254) + .8 \times 0$$

$$= -0.80$$

$$\hat{y}_3 \quad = (D_2 + R_2) \times S_{3-4}$$

$$= (1250 - .80) \times 1$$

$$= 1249.2$$

These values are shown in the second row of Table 11.4.

The calculations for the third and fourth quarter of the first year (1969) and for the first quarter of the next year (1970) use initial values of the seasonal factor. The first set of calculations that incorporate only values based on previous experience is the second quarter of 1970, the sixth quarter for which data has been recorded (in monthly data, this would correspond to the second month of the second year or 14th month recorded). To illustrate, we show the calculations for the sixth row of Table 11.4.

In 1970, $y_2 = 1275$. With $\gamma = .2$ as before

$$D_2 = .2(y_2/S_{2-4}) + .8(D_1 + R_1)$$

$$= .2 \times 1275/0.9989 + .8 \times (1287.0 + 5.38)$$

$$= 1289.2$$

$$S_2 = .2(y_2/D_2) + .8\, S_{2-4}$$

$$= .2 \times 1275/1289.2 + .8 \times .9989$$

$$= 0.9969$$

$$R_2 = .2(D_2 - D_1) + .8\, R_1$$

$$= .2(1289.2 - 1287.0) + .8 \times 5.38$$

$$= 4.74$$

Table 11.4. Number of office visits (y_t) to a given dentist by quarter and extended forecasting calculations

Year	Quarter	y_t	S_1	S_2	S_3	S_4	D	R	$\hat{y}_{t+1}$
1969	1	1254	1.0000	1.0000	1.0000	1.0000	1254.0	0.0	1254.0
	2	1234		.9974			1250.0	−0.8	1249.2
	3	1300			1.0065		1259.4	1.2	1260.6
	4	1373				1.0140	1283.1	5.7	1288.8
1970	1	1280	.9989				1287.0	5.4	1289.1
	2	1275		.9969			1289.2	4.8	1302.4
	3	1320			1.0086		1297.8	5.5	1321.6
	4	1384				1.0216	1315.6	8.0	1322.1
1971	1	1310	.9974				1321.2	7.5	1322.9
	2	1295		.9923			1323.0	6.4	1340.8
	3	1330			1.0073		1327.2	5.9	1362.0
	4	1485				1.0361	1357.3	10.7	1364.5
1972	1	1460	1.0085				1387.1	14.6	1390.9
	2	1250		.9959			1373.3	8.9	1392.2
	3	1275				.9935	1358.9	4.2	1412.4
	4	1394				1.0340	1359.6	3.5	1374.7
1973	1	1286	.9979				1345.5	0.0	1313.1
	2	1299		.9742			1342.7	−0.6	1333.3
	3	1360				.9966	1347.5	0.5	1393.7
	4	1370				1.0311	1343.4	−0.4	1340.2
1974	1	1368	1.0012				1348.5	0.7	1314.5
	2	1350		.9784			1356.5	2.2	1354.1
	3	1428			1.0053		1373.5	5.1	1421.6
	4	1465				1.0361	1387.1	6.8	1395.6
1975	1	1393	1.0009				1393.4	6.7	1369.8
	2	1380		.9796			1402.2	7.1	1416.7
	3	1440			1.0079		1413.9	8.1	1473.4
	4	1498				1.0389	1426.7	9.0	1437.1
1976	1	1490	1.0068				1446.3	11.1	1427.7
	2	1398		.9763			1451.4	9.9	1472.8
	3	1460			1.0065		1458.7	9.4	1525.3
	4	1520				1.0383	1467.1	9.2	1486.3

From R. L. Burford, 1970, *Basic Statistics for Business and Economics,* Charles E. Merrill, Columbus, Ohio, Figure 16.1, p. 441. Reprinted by permission of the author.

$$\hat{y}_3 = (D_2 + R_2) \cdot S_{3-4}$$

$$= (1289.2 + 4.74) \times 1.0065$$

$$= 1302.4$$

Table 11.4 shows the values of the seasonal factors $S_1, S_2, S_3,$ and S_4, which are updated after every four quarters. These show that the fourth quarter is high and the second quarter (generally)

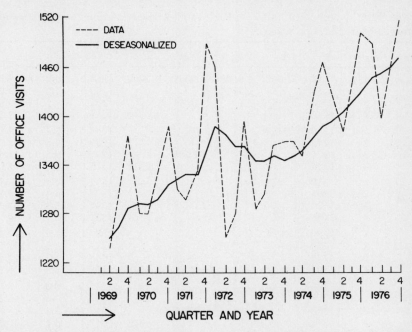

Figure 11.4. Graph of deseasonalized values against the observed time series given in Table 11.4.

low in terms of the dentist's workload. The column headed D contains the deseasonalized or smoothed values of the series. These values are seen to increase steadily until 1972, when they oscillate and then continue to increase to the end of the period. In Figure 11.4 the deseasonalized values are plotted, together with the original series, against time to show the smoothing effect. Figure 11.5 shows the predicted values plotted against the observed time series. Notice that the predicted values in Figure 11.5 are less variable about the trend than are the original series, although these predicted values still show seasonal variations. Finally, to measure the accuracy of the prediction, we compare the correlation of $\hat{y}_t$ and y_t against the serial correlation of the series. We have for 30 pairs of observations

Serial correlation of y_t with $y_{t+1} = .52$

Correlation of y_t with $\hat{y}_t = .65$.

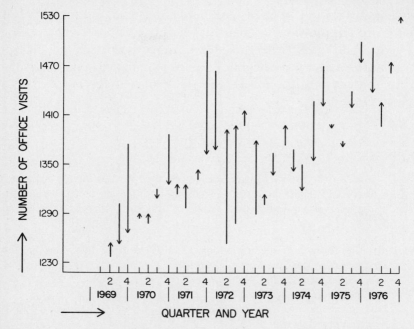

Figure 11.5. Graph showing deviations of predicted value from actual value.

As in multiple regression, we can interpret the difference of these correlations squared as the percent improvement due to the prediction. In this case, this is $(.65^2 - .52^2) = .1521 = .15\%$.

In general, we cannot expect much stability of our estimates or accuracy of our forecasts in the first four to six years. One's ability to predict the future increases with the amount of past records. The information in past records for prediction is, however, self-limiting, since, as the series progresses, the components of the time series will also change and may not in fact be mutually independent as we have assumed. The approach given here (extended forecasting) is responsive to shifts in the time series, being more responsive to changes for higher values of γ. No forecast based on past data can predict an abrupt change in the time series unless other concomitant information is also considered. Forecasts tend to lag behind new departures in a time series. Decisions based on automatic forecasting procedures should not therefore be crucial. If the cost of a poor decision is high, then all ancillary information should be used, preferably in a valid causal model. If causes are unknown or unquantifiable, it is often preferable to use an "educated" guess when a sudden change is anticipated. In this way the forecaster can integrate his past experience and knowledge of the system with the presumed effects of new factors, such as a change in the law.

EXERCISES

(*Note.* Some of the following exercises in extended forecasting are computationally heavy and might justify the development of a computer program. An S.A.S. program for extended forecasting of quarterly records is given in Section 12.6).

11.1 In the following, specify which variable is more likely to be the independent (i.e., predictor) variable:
   a) degree of disability and income
   b) height and weight
   c) statewide mortality rate and number of hospital beds per 1000 of the population
   d) prevalence of iatrogenic disease and average number of office visits per doctor
   e) vital capacity and age.

11.2 a) To express the fact that a regression line

$$\hat{y} = a + b$$

passes through the joint mean $(\bar{x}, \bar{y})$ the regression equation is sometimes written

$$(\hat{y} - \bar{y}) = b(x - \bar{x}).$$

From the equivalence of these two equations, derive an expression for a in terms of b, $\bar{x}$, and $\bar{y}$.
   b) Likewise, the multiple regression

$$y = a + bx + cz$$

may be expressed as

$$\hat{y} - \bar{y} = b(x - \bar{x}) + c(z - \bar{z}).$$

Find the expression for a in terms of b, c, $\bar{x}$, $\bar{y}$, and $\bar{z}$.

11.3 Laboratory expenses (y) in dollars per month and laboratory revenue (x) in dollars per month were collected for a group practice over a year (12 months). The mean monthly expense and mean monthly revenue were \$224.75 and \$316.67, respectively. The correlation coefficient between monthly expenses and revenue was 0.988. The standard deviation for expenses and revenue were \$34.35 and \$55.83, respectively.

a) From this information, test whether the correlation coefficient is significantly different from zero (at the 5% level).
b) If so, then derive the linear regression equation. (Use the formulas $b = r\, s_y/s_x$ and $a = \bar{y} - b\bar{x}$.)
c) Then, state on the average how much of each additional dollar in revenue goes into the expense of running the laboratory.
d) What is the overhead? (What is the expense of having the laboratory if there is no revenue?)
e) What is the break even point? (What is the minimum monthly revenue required to cover overhead in an average month?)

11.4 We wish to investigate the time that the professional nurse devotes to direct patient care. The factors expected to affect this time are the size of the professional staff, the size of the non-professional nursing staff, the general condition of patients, and the size of the nursing unit. Write down the form of the regression equation you would use in this study and define its terms.

11.5 Plotting the number of hospital admissions in a year against the number of available beds in each of 51 states reveals that both California and New York are outliers. Data for these two states were omitted and regressions calculated as shown in Table 11.5.

a) Test whether for each year the quadratic regression adds significantly to the proportion of the variation explained by a linear regression (use tables of F at the 5% level).
b) Table 11.2 gives, for Virginia, the actual number of beds and admissions for 1969 and 1970. Using the linear regression coefficients of Table 11.5, which are based on 49 states, calculate the expected number of admissions in Virginia
   1) in 1969, using the 1969 linear regression,
   2) in 1969, using the 1970 linear regression,
   3) in 1970, using the 1969 linear regression,
   4) in 1970, using the 1970 linear regression.
c) In order to compare these estimates with the corresponding estimates based on linear regressions derived from all 50 states, divide your answers in 5(b) by the actual number of admissions in that year and compare these ratios with those given in Table 11.2. Which set of data (the original 50 states or those omitting California and New York) give the better estimates for Virginia?

11.6 Give two examples of a simple (i.e., univariate) time series and two examples of a complex (i.e., multivariate) time series.

Table 11.5. The amount of variation explained (R^2) and the coefficients of different regression models fitted to 1969 and 1970 date on admissions (y) and hospital beds (x) omitting California and New York

	1969			
	R^2	a	b	c
$\hat{y} = a + bx$	93.6%	51,907	19.55	–
$\hat{y} = a + bx + cx^2$	93.8%	22,341	22.48	−0.00004
	1970			
	R^2	a	b	c
$\hat{y} = a + bx$	94.3%	50,762	20.59	–
$\hat{y} = a + bx + cx^2$	94.5%	20,600	23.63	−0.00004

Source: *Hospitals* (1970) 44(2):501 and *Hospitals* (1971) 45(2):490.

11.7 A friend insists that the time series given in column y_t in Table 11.4, the number of quarterly visits to a dentist, has in fact been created by a random number generator on a computer. Test this series for randomness using both procedures given in Section 11.10.

11.8 Calculate moving averages for the quarterly data given in Table 11.4 using the expression

Moving average at $t = (y_{t-2} + 2y_{t-1} + 2y_t + 2y_{t+1} + y_{t+2})/8$

and compare this with an exponentially smoothed series derived from y_t in Table 11.4 using $\gamma = .2$

$$\hat{y}_{t+1} = \gamma \cdot y_t + (1 - \gamma)\hat{y}_t$$

11.9 The number of deliveries, omitting inductions, in an obstetric unit is given for each 12-hour period in a week. This time series was 6, 9, 8, 11, 7, 10, 6, 12, 9, 12, 10, 13, 12, 15. Apply extended forecasting formulas to this data and forecast the number of deliveries expected in the next two 12-hour periods after the end of the current series. (Use a value of $\gamma = .3$ in these calculations.) *Note.* D, S_1, S_2, and R are 6, 1, 1, and 0, respectively, for the first observation.)

11.10 Repeat the above exercise with $\gamma = .1$. This will illustrate the effect of different values of γ on the predictions.

11.11 Given that y is equal to the percentage of the Gross National Product that is spent on health care in the United States, past annual data has been used to deduce the trend line

$$y = a + b \cdot t$$

where t = year, $a = -387$, $b = 0.2$.

(This exercise illustrates that date or year can be used as a regression variable.)

a) Show that the predicted value in 1975 is 8%.

b) By what year will the proportion of the GNP spent on health care reach 15%?

LITERATURE CITED

Brooks, G. H., and H. L. Beenhakker. 1964. A new technique for prediction of future hospital bed needs. Hosp. Manag. 97:47–50.

Brown, R. G. 1963. Smoothing, Forcasting and Prediction. Prentice-Hall Inc., Englewood Cliffs, New Jersey.

Commission on Hospital Care. 1957. Hospital Care in the U.S. Harvard University Press, Cambridge, Mass., p. 272.

Donabedian, A. 1973. Aspects of Medical Care Administration. Harvard University Press, Cambridge, Mass., p. 454, 463.

Fleiss, P. 1973. Statistical Methods for Rates and Proportions. John Wiley & Sons Inc., New York.

Froggatt, P., M. Y. Dudgeon, and J. D. Merritt. 1969. Consultations in general practice: Analysis of individual frequencies. Brit. Prev. J. Soc. Med. 23:1.

Galbraith, J. K. 1972. The New Industrial State. 2nd Ed. André Deutsch Ltd., London.

Jelinek, R. C. 1967. A structural model for the patient care operation. Health Serv. Res. 2:226–242.

Kempthorne, O. 1952. The Design and Analysis of Experiments. John Wiley & Sons Inc., New York, p. 43.

Kendall, M. G. 1973. Time Series. Charles Griffin & Co. Ltd., London, Appendix A.

Peacock, J. B., M. Goodman, S. J. Kilpatrick and G. Sumner. Morbidity on a new housing estate. Soc. Sci. Med. (In press.)

Phillip, P. J. 1970. On exponential smoothing: An extension. Health Serv. Res. 5:372–377.

Susser, M. 1973. Causal Thinking in the Health Sciences. Oxford University Press, London, p. 60.

FURTHER READING

Anderson, R., B. Smedby, and B. Eklund. 1971. Automatic interaction detection program for analyzing health survey data. Health Serv. Res. 6(2):165–183. (An alternative to regression analysis.)

Draper, N. R., and H. Smith. 1966. Applied Regression Analysis. John Wiley & Sons, Inc., New York. (Chapter 9, Multiple regression applied to analysis of variance problems—an elementary matrix treatment.)

Hamburg, M. 1970. Statistical Analysis for Decision Making. Harcourt, Brace & Co., New York. (See Section 11.4, "The fitting of trend lines by the method of least squares for a detailed account of using linear and quadratic regression to fit trend lines to economic time series.")

Kilpatrick, S. J. 1975. Factors in morbidity. Soc. Sci. Med. 9:319–325. (Graphs of R^2.)

McLain, J. O. 1971. Exponential smoothing: Appropriate and inappropriate applications. Health Serv. Res. 6:256–259.

McLaughlin, C. P., and A. Sheldon. 1974. The Future and Medical Care: A Health Manager's Guide to Forecasting. Ballinger, Cambridge, Mass. (Describes the Delphi technique.)

Quenouille, M. H. 1966. Introductory Statistics. Pergamon Press Ltd., Oxford. (Chapter 8 for transformations.)

Robinson, E. A. 1967. Multichannel Time Series Analysis with Digital Computer Programs. Holden-Day Inc., San Francisco.

Schweder, T. 1971. The precision of population projections studied by multiple prediction methods. Demography 8(4):441. (For population experts only, difficult matrix notation.)

Searle, S. R. 1975. "Some Unifying Thoughts on the Analysis of Variance." Paper read at A.S.A. meeting, Atlanta. (Equivalence of analyses of variance and regression.)

Shain, M., and M. I. Roemer. 1959. Hospital costs relate to the supply of beds. Mod. Hosp. 92:71.

Shiskin, J. 1967. The X-11 Variant of the Census Method II Seasonal Adjustment Program. Technical Paper #15, U.S. Bureau of the Census.

Sposato, D. P., and A. H. Spinner. 1970. Forecasting by a modified exponential smoothing method. Health Serv. Res. 5:141–147.

12

Role of the Computer in Health Care Administration and Research

12.1 INTRODUCTION

In addition to having a background knowledge of statistical principles and decision making, the health care administrator should understand the basic principles of the computer. The **digital computer** has rapidly become a major tool of the quantitatively oriented administrator and researcher. To use it properly and to integrate it optimally into a health care facility, one should thoroughly review the information system and its objectives. Too often, the introduction of a computer without prior planning merely exaggerates the faults of the original information system. Also, since the decision to automate some aspects of health care records is generally irreversible, the organization will have to live with a poor information system until the next upgrading of computers (which in itself may be precipitated by a bad initial choice). Paradoxically, the best decision is often to stay with the existing procedures rather than to embark on an expensive and irreversible path toward computerization. Delaying until the "bugs" are ironed out of the computer system may save money and, more importantly, the good will of the health care professionals, who will interact with the computer. Too often, naive managers have been "oversold" on the virtues of a computer system by aggressive computer salesmen.

Basically, computing machinery may be centralized into one

233

large machine that will serve all purposes, or diversified into small computers dedicated to specific tasks. Professional computer managers prefer the centralization of machines and justify this preference in terms of efficiency and reduced costs. While these reasons may apply to the best organized and managed central facilities, centralization can also result in a badly organized and managed computer system that forces management to use the computer in ways that are possible rather than in ways that are desirable.

The alternative method, that of allowing units of the organization with clear-cut computer needs to meet these needs themselves, tends to develop competition rather than collaboration among the staffs of these smaller systems. This may mean that personnel are inflexible, and that it may take more people to discharge the total computer needs of the organization than it would in a centralized shop. The diversified arrangement of specialized computers, however, is easier to fit into an overall administrative structure and will allow for changes and modifications in the separate components more easily than the centralized computer facility will.

In summary, the use of computers in an organization may range from being highly centralized to being highly diversified. In the centralized case, the machinery is relatively fixed but the personnel are flexible and may be redirected to different tasks. In the case of diversified and specialized equipment, the personnel are relatively inflexible both administratively and professionally, but the machinery is more flexible, allowing for growth, curtailment, and changes. In many large health care facilities (especially those with educational, training, and research roles) the approach is to allow for both a major centralized computer facility and separate computer facilities dedicated to specific roles (such as the automation of the clinical laboratory).

12.2 PRINCIPLES OF COMPUTING

12.2.1 Computer Operations

Administrators and research workers who depend on the computer should know what a computer can and cannot do. A computer can do arithmetic; that is, it can add and subtract and therefore it can multiply and divide (by repeated addition or subtraction). It can perform basic logical operations, since it can compare two numbers and indicate which is greater. Computers execute a series of commands (a program), which reduces to adding, subtracting, comparing, and relocating numbers in different addresses, i.e., parts of its "memory." The computer's ability to compare numbers enables workers to use programs with conditional branches, instructing the computer to follow one sequence of instructions rather than another under certain conditions. This also enables us to make a computer repeat a calculation, etc., until some condition is met. In iterative computing, the whole process is repeated until the "best" result is found.

Finally we may communicate with the computer through a variety of input/output devices: cards, tape, keyboard, light-sensitive pen; printer, plotter, cathode ray tube—by reading in instructions and data and getting back results or error messages. The languages by which computers are programmed are rarely those in which the computer operates. Considerable effort has been spent in devising programming languages as close to the spoken word as possible. These languages are typified by COBOL (*Co*mmon *B*usiness *O*riented *L*anguage) and FORTRAN (*For*mula *Trans*lation). As the names suggest, these are designed for business applications and scientific computing, respectively. The computer is equipped with compliers (conversion routines), which translate these higher level languages into machine language.

12.2.2 Properties of Computers

The most important asset of a digital computer is its speed. It performs its operations extremely quickly (about one million times faster than man). Moreover, computers are becoming faster, allowing for considerable trade-off between speed and convenience. Recent developments, as a result, are interactive computing and time sharing, in which many customers use one machine simultaneously. In fact, the modern computer is so fast that while it is reading in the statements and data of one program it may be performing another's calculations. This exploits the fact that input/output devices are much slower than the internal machine speeds so that a computer is almost idle internally when it is only "reading" or "writing" (as communications with the computer are called). In summary, computers are very fast, and as they become faster it is possible to make them more accessible by requiring them to do more interpreting or translating from human terms to machine terms. (It is conceivable that in the future we will talk to computers and they will reply, asking for further specification of our commands.)

Clearly, this immense speed would be useless without a very high level of dependability. Computers break down, but rarely, and when they do, it is all too obvious, since no results are produced. Errors can also occur in the output, but this is invariably due to an error in the programs being used or to the input data. Occasionally, the output printer will malfunction. Such errors are often difficult to detect. A good rule of thumb is to compare the results against your best judgment of what the results should have been. If these are divergent, ask the operator to run a similar (test) problem for which you know the answer, or check the data input, the program, and your expectation. Sometimes it is best to repeat the whole job from scratch to find the source of error, or someone else can be asked to repeat the job using the same machine. One must remember that errors are made by people much more frequently than by computers.

12.2.3 Functions of Computers

From an operational viewpoint, computers are used in data processing, calculations, or simulations. In data processing, emphasis is placed on the ability of the computer to repeat a relatively simple procedure quickly and without error. These types of jobs usually involve reading and writing with a minimum of calculation. For example, the reading, reordering, and listing of patients' names in alphabetical order would be a typical data processing job, as would be the billing of patients discharged from the hospital or the maintenance of an inventory of the pharmacy. In calculating, emphasis is placed on the arithmetic function of the system. Typically, the machine sits humming to itself, and after many long, repeated, and often complex calculations may print out a simple number as the answer. In a simulation a mathematical description of a system is programmed, and the computer calculates the outcome of different starting values, or of running the system repetitively a large number of times. Usually, there is a chance element in the system and consequently in its mathematical description. Repeated runs are made to find the typical behavior of the system and to find its limits under the assumptions of the model. The classic simulation in health care is the simulation of an epidemic among a population of susceptibles. While theory predicts what will happen if certain rates of infection are assumed, the computer simulation predicts what might happen if chance movements of the population result in infection rates varying about this assumed rate (Bailey, 1957). Similarly, models of outpatient emergency clinics can be developed which will predict the range of waiting times of patients.

12.3   COMPUTERS IN HEALTH CARE TRAINING

In addition to being used in Computer Assisted Instruction and in testing by means of multiple choice questions (Kilpatrick, 1971), the computer can be used directly in training health care professionals and health care administrators. Commerical airlines use complex airplane simulators as a part of the training of pilots in flying new aircraft. The justification of this is that it is cheaper to run a simulator than an aircraft with no pay load. Also, the possible loss of capital and life, if the student pilot crashes, is avoided. The Pentagon uses war games to train officers in military strategy. Again, this is cheaper than the cost of a full-scale exercise and avoids the risk to human life. Business students play business games with different teams managing hypothetical companies with assumed assets and types of products. In all of these examples, computers are used to calculate the likely outcome of a decision based on a simulation model.

The computer can be similarly used in health care. In training health care administrators, a model of the particular system they will direct can be created and the student can be presented with various contingencies and asked to make certain decisions. In a short time the student can gain a useful background of experience in coping with problems (albeit in an artificial setting) frequently recurring in a hospital, group practice, department of nursing, or public health district. One advantage of the computer model is that the student and his teachers are forced to develop criteria by which to evaluate decisions.

The same approach could be taken to the training of health care personnel. Physicians learn the art of diagnosis and treatment by attending clinico-pathological conferences and by trial and error, first in training and then in practice. The expense of medical education would be lessened, and the quality of the finished product improved by the use of computer simulations of diagnostic procedures. This has been reported (Feurzeig et al., 1964), using the Socratic method, and research is underway for the use of a mannikin which would simulate some of the signs of various conditions, including reactions to treatment.

12.4   COMPUTERS IN HEALTH CARE

There are great conceptual similarities between computer programs that simulate a patient and those programs that are used to give differential diagnoses based on data from actual patients. In other words, the relationship between disease processes and their signs and symptoms is needed in both types of program. In computer diagnosis, the output usually contains a list of potential diagnoses ranked in decreasing order of likelihood (sometimes with an associated probability).

The universality of such programs, however, is reduced by the location of the physician who wants to use the system. A medical student, an intern on a pediatric service, a specialist in otology, say, will have different prior probabilities of seeing a child with tinnitus. As we have seen earlier, these prior probabilities affect the posterior or calculated probability. A similar approach could be taken in the diagnosis and treatment of patients by computer. Some general papers have been written in this area (Ledley, 1967) but clearly this application is in its earliest stages.

More direct use of computers in health care is in the clinical laboratory, where the computer is an established component of automated clinical chemistry (Krieg et al., 1971; Westlake and Bennington, 1972).

The data processing aspects of the computer can be used in multiphasic screening, where many individuals undergo routine but comprehensive physical examinations that are largely automated. Here the function of the computer is to collate information from the different test values and to print a uniform report for the physician to review before he sees the patient. Potentially, the computer in multiphasic screening would also compare an individual's current test values against his past results and indicate where significant changes had occurred since the last examination. This longitudinal approach, which uses each individual as his own norm, should be more informative than the current practice of evaluating a patient's vital signs against norms from a distribution of presumably healthy individuals.

The computer can, of course, be wired directly to the patient, sampling and analyzing EKG and EEG patterns, pulse rate, temperature, etc. Clearly, this is only feasible or necessary when the patient is critically ill and under intensive care. The computer can be programmed to screen the vital signs of the patient to alert the medical staff when there is a deterioration in the patient's condition. As in multiphasic screening, the patient's own past history can be used to establish base lines determining whether he is getting better or worse. Combinations of changes that independently mean little but together are suggestive of a forthcoming attack can likewise be recognized by the computer. Finally, research has been conducted on the prediction of crises, using repeatedly sampled readings from a critically ill patient (Wilson, 1970).

12.5 COMPUTERS IN HEALTH CARE ADMINISTRATION

The uses of computers in hospitals range from the unit record of transactions, which must legally be recorded, to the summary tables designed to give the hospital director information on the operation of the hospital. The dilemma arising here is that if the summary tables are produced as a by-product of basic records, the consequent delay before they are available renders them of little value. One approach is to prepare data independently for current summary tables. This service may be contracted for, through PAS (Professional Activity Study) and MAP (Medical Audit Program). PAS and MAP are supported chiefly by the participating hospitals. The hospitals are required to report the data on their patients, recorded systematically in a standard manner. The data are scrutinized and processed by computer, and the information is returned in such a format that each hospital obtains an overall view of its activities, as well as details regarding individual patients. This collection of information is much more quickly available and comprehensible than the original records.

A similar service is provided by the HAS (Hospital Administration Services) program. HAS participants report monthly values of various general, departmental, and related indicators or indices for various services that the hospital provides. These reports are collated and summarized according to the size of the hospital. The distribution of the values of each indicator in a given month is given by quartiles along with the participating hospital's own performance. In this way, the administrator can compare his hospital's record with the records of similar hospitals. Other aspects of the HAS program are its Spotlight reports, six-month national reports, departmental performance charts, and productivity and cost analyses.

It is relevant to ask how accurate these summaries must be. Thus, Glaser (1971), in discussing health information systems, states that "much machinery, effort and expense continues to be devoted to looking at all the items of interest routinely, when in fact a sample would be adequate." If complete accuracy is required, some such scheme involving abstracts on all patients' records is necessary. However, if the participating administrator simply wants assurance that no large change, in costs, for example, has occurred, sampling is indicated. Television coverage of elections has made the public aware of how accurate small samples can be in predicting the outcome of an election. By the same token, administrators should ask whether the information from, say, a 5% sample would not provide the information he requires (at one twentieth of the cost). Biases in the predictions could probably be allowed for by the use of regression techniques.

A chronicle of common misuses of computers in administration would include this tendency to ask for complete information on all aspects of the hospital's administration simply because the computer can produce it. Such a request soon results in thousands of pages of computer output that no one ever looks at even though they may be faithfully distributed to various levels of administration. Instead, the computer should be programmed to screen information against pre-established limits and its output should be limited to exception statistics, i.e., those tables or records in which, according to some criterion, the usual range has been exceeded. Finally, figures lie—not perhaps in themselves, but in the interpretation placed on them by the untutored (Mainland, 1968).

12.6 COMPUTERS IN RESEARCH

The introduction of modern computing facilities has revolutionized the practice of statistics in the recent past. Most obviously, the advent of the computer has removed the sometimes excessive drudgery of statistical calculations and permits the use of more complex procedures, heretofore considered impractical because of the labor in calculating. It follows therefore that all applied statisticians and most research workers who use statistics have to learn how to use their local computational facilities. Once this barrier to the use of the computer has been overcome, the investigator will find that he is using the computer facility for all but the most trivial of his statistical calculations.

In the last ten years, computer installations have tended to increase in size and in speed and to serve many different types of applications via remote terminals. The computer industry has used this increase in complexity to make the computer more easily accessible to the unsophisticated user. For example, programming languages such as FORTRAN, ALGOL, or APL already are partially oriented to the way we think and use algebra. More recently, large computer installations offer their users access to a variety of packaged statistical programs. These are all collections of standard statistical procedures. Many are available today and an interested reader should inquire about which set of packaged programs is available to him at his local computer facility. The most commonly available are BMD (Dixon, 1975), SPSS (Nie et al., 1975) and SAS 72 (Barr et al., 1972).

Although each package of statistical programs differs from every other set of statistical programs, the flavor can perhaps be best learned from an example. The following section describes the use of SAS 72 in completing some of the examples or exercises used elsewhere in this text.

SAS (Statistical Analysis System) is based on the assumption that the investigator will want to analyze multiple readings repeated on a series of different units. Thus, in Chapter 11 we analyzed the number of admissions and the number of hospital beds in 1969 in each of 50 states. Here each state is defined as a unit and the number of admissions and beds as the readings.

SAS also assumes that the investigator will want to modify his data and to generate other data from the original observations. To permit this, SAS constructs data sets on command.

SAS is format-free. The user does not have to specify the layout of tables, etc. If desired, he may insert titles by adding a card of the form:

TITLE   'Write title here

Note that a semi-colon (;) is used to end all statements within the body of the SAS program. Data cards and the MACRO statement are the only exceptions.

Finally, an SAS program must start and end with certain job control cards (JCL). As an example, the cards used to read in and to print out our data on hospital admissions and beds are shown using the 1972 version of SAS:

```
//EXAMPLE JOB (7323,HB09), SMITH
//EXEC SAS
//SAS.SYSIN DD*
TITLE 'REFERENCE HOSPITALS 1970 VOL 44 PAGE 501';
DATA;
INPUT BEDS 1-8 ADMISSIONS 9-17;
CARDS;
```

```
        179785              2405840
        115534              2557930
          .                   .
          .                   .
          .                   .
         28049               715417
          3151               63105
```

PROCEDURE PRINT;

//

Each line above represents a card that is keypunched and read into the computer. The first three and the last are job control cards. The first card says that a job called "example" is to be processed and charged to Smith, whose programmer number is 7323 and whose department code is HB09. The second card informs the computer that SAS is to be used. The third card prepares SAS for action. The last card tells the computer that input has ended and starts the computer processing the job.

TITLE 'REFERENCE HOSPITALS 1970 VOL 44 PAGE 501';

This title card will cause the reference to be used as a heading on each page of the output until a subsequent title occurs.

DATA;

This data card initiates the creation of a data set into which the data will be read.

INPUT BEDS 1–8 ADMISSIONS 9–17;

This input card informs the computer that columns one to eight of each data card will contain a number that is the number of beds in that state and that columns nine to seventeen will contain the number of admissions. These two variables are called "Beds" and "Admiss," respectively, the latter being an abbreviation of "admissions," since variable names in SAS cannot be more than eight characters long.

CARDS;

This card tells the computer that the following information is to be considered as data. Note that these cards do not end in semi-colons. After these cards have been read in, the computer has in its memory a data set consisting of 51 pairs of readings called Beds and Admiss.

PROCEDURE PRINT;

This tells the computer what to do with the data set. Here the print procedure is used so that the data is simply printed out in an unchanged form as follows:

REFERENCE HOSPITALS 1970 VOL 44 PAGE 501

BEDS	ADMISSIONS
179785	2405840
115534	2557930
.	.
.	.
.	.
28049	715417
3151	63105

This, of course, is an over-simplified example. We have simply passed information through a computer and listed it in an unchanged form. The analytical power of SAS is contained in its procedure statements. These, in effect, apply the named statistical procedure to the data. The list of procedures available is:

PRINT, SORT, RANK, PLOT, MEANS, REGR, RSQUARE, STEPWISE, ANOVA, DUNCAN, NESTED, LATTICE, RQUE, CANCORR, DISCRIM, FACTOR, CORR, SPEARMAN, FREQ, GUTTMAN, PLAN.

By inserting a card

PROCEDURE PLOT;

a scatter diagram of 51 points will be printed. The scaling is done automatically and the names of the variables are printed on the axes.

PROCEDURE MEANS;

This card will cause all of the standard statistics to be calculated and printed for each variable: the number of observations, the standard deviation, the range and the coefficient of variation.

PROCEDURE REGR;

This card is used for regression analysis. In addition, one must also specify the form of the regression equation to be used. Here we are interested in the regression of the number of admissions on the number of beds and so we insert the card:

MODEL ADMISS = BEDS/PREDICTED;

This card tells the computer that the simple linear regression:

Admissions = $a + b$ Beds

is intended and causes a predicted number of admissions to be calculated for each state from the regression equation. The output for an SAS program prints the program statements which have been input as well as the results. A typical output is shown below, listing the SAS statements on the right side of the page.

TITLE 'REFERENCE HOSPITALS 1970 VOL 44 P501';
DATA;
INPUT BEDS 1−8 ADMISS 9−17;
CARDS;
179785   2405840
115534   2557930
.
.
.
28049   715417
3151   63105
PROCEDURE PRINT;
TITLE 'EXAMPLE OF SAS';

EXAMPLE OF SAS

OBS	BEDS	ADMISS
1	179785	2405840
2	115534	2557930
.	.	.
.	.	.
.	.	.
50	28049	715417
51	3151	63105

PROCEDURE PLOT;
TITLE 'EXAMPLE OF SAS';

EXAMPLE OF SAS

PLOT OF BEDS vs ADMISS

BEDS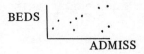

ADMISS

PROCEDURE MEANS;
TITLE 'EXAMPLE OF SAS';

EXAMPLE OF SAS

VARIABLE	N	MEAN	STD. DEV	...	LOW	HIGH
BEDS	51	27505	33150	...	1819	179785
ADMISS	51	571784	581964	...	43515	2557930

PROCEDURE REGR;
MODEL ADMISS = BEDS / PREDICTED;
TITLE 'EXAMPLE OF SAS';

EXAMPLE OF SAS

SOURCE	DF	SUM OF SQUARES	MEAN SQUARE	F
Regression	1	15379×10^9	15379×10^9	481
Error	49	1555×10^9	32×10^9	
Total	50	16934×10^9		

PROB OF F 0.0001

R-Square = 0.91

SOURCE	B VALUES
Intercept	111619
BEDS	16.73

OBS	OBSERVED	PREDICTED	RESIDUAL
1	2405840	3119407	−173567
2	2557930	2044493	513436
.			
.			
.			
.			
.			
.			
.			
50	715417	580876	134540
51	63105	164334	−101229

If, from an examination of the plot of admissions against beds on the residuals between the predicted and observed values, you want to apply a quadratic regression

$$\text{Admissions} = a + b \text{ Beds} + c \text{ (Beds)}^2$$

then all that is needed is to replace the model card with

MODEL ADMISS = BEDS BEDSSQ;

where BEDSSQ is the name of a variable generated by

BEDSSQ = BEDS * BEDS;

i.e., the square of the number of beds.

Note that in order to keep the above descriptions as simple as possible many optimal features of SAS have been omitted. It is important, however, to realize that one can also program in SAS, using this package to take care of input, output, and format details. An example of programming a calculation in SAS is an exponential smoothing of a time series. The program is as follows, omitting the JCL cards:

```
DATA;
INPUT Y 1 - 10;
N = N+ 1;
IF N = 1 THEN RETURN;
IF N = 2 THEN SMOOTH = 1254;
SMOOTH = .2 * Y + .8 * SMOOTH;
CARDS;
1254
1234
    .
    .
    .

PROCEDURE PRINT;
//
```

This set of instructions will create a data set, will read the time series y_t into it from the first 10 columns of the data cards, and, as each card is read, will also generate a second variable 'smooth' that will be the exponential smoothed average of the series. Note that a count is kept of the cards read since N is increased by 1 for each card. The only purpose that N serves is to start the exponential smoothing off properly. After the first card is read

$$Y = 1254, N = 1$$

and the computer skips the remaining statements to read a second card. Now

$$Y = 1234, N = 2 \text{ and so SMOOTH} = 1254$$

and therefore SMOOTH is evaluated as $.2 \times 1234 + .8 \times 1254 = 1250$. For the third and subsequent cards, the value of N is immaterial.

To calculate the moving average

$$\text{M.A.} = (y_{t-3} + 2y_{t-2} + 2y_{t-1} + y_t)/6$$

for a simple time series in SAS one would use:

```
DATA;
INPUT Y 1-2;
N = N + 1;
T3 = T2;
T2 = T1;
T1 = T;
T = Y;
MA = (T3 + 2 * T2 + 2 * T1 + T)/6;
CARDS;
  6
  9
  8
 11
  .
  .
  .
```

The data set will be as follows:

OBS	Y	N	T3	T2	T1	T	MA
1	6	1	0	0	0	6	1.0
2	9	2	0	0	6	9	3.5
3	8	3	0	6	9	8	6.3
4	11	4	6	9	8	11	8.5
etc.							

Note that this moving average is not defined until the fourth observation has been read. Note also that all variables are initially zero.

The SAS program for the extended forecasting calculations described in Chapter 11 now follows:

```
TITLE    'EXTENDED FORECASTING FOR QUARTERLY DATA';
DATA;
INPUT Y 1-6;
A = .2; B = .2; C = .2;                                    ... (a)
AA = 1 − A; BB = 1 − B; CC = 1 − C;
ZZ = YY;
IF   I = 0 THEN D = Y;
IF   I > 0 THEN GO TO J1;
SS = 1; SSS = 1;
S1 = 1; S2 = 1; S3 = 1; S4 = 1;
J1:  IF I = 1 THEN   SS = S2;
IF   I = 1     THEN SSS = S3;
IF   I = 2     THEN  SS = S3;
IF   I = 2     THEN SSS = S4;
IF   I = 3     THEN  SS = S4;
IF   I = 3     THEN SSS = S1;
IF   I = 4     THEN  SS = S1;
IF   I = 4     THEN SSS = S2;
DD = D;
  D = (A * Y/SS) + (AA * (D + R));
  S = (B * Y/D) + (BB * SS);
  R = (C * (D−DD)) + (CC * R);
YY = (D + R) * SSS;
  I = I + 1;
IF      I = 5     THEN I = 1;
IF      I = 1     THEN S1 = S;
IF      I = 2     THEN S2 = S;
IF      I = 3     THEN S3 = S;
IF      I = 4     THEN S4 = S;
CARDS;
```

  .
  .
  .

This program is clearly cumbersome and could be made more elegant if desired. The program demonstrates the (current) limitation of SAS in that one cannot easily program cycles (DO loops in

FORTRAN). The equivalent FORTRAN program would be much simpler.

This program may easily be modified to monthly or other data by adding to or removing from the IF statements that run from IF I = 1 to IF I = 4 and IF I = 5.

Note that one can easily change the values of A, B, C in card (a) in order to improve the fit of the predicted value YY to Y. There is no need for A=B=C except for computational simplicity. Different values can be tried provided that the values of A, B, C lie between 0 and 1. D, S, R and YY are the deseasonalized values, seasonal factors, trend values, and forecast respectively. It is a simple matter in SAS to plot the calculated values and to apply other statistical techniques to them to investigate the goodness of fit between the observed and predicted time series.

A major revision of SAS known as SAS 76 has just been released (Barr et al., 1976). This version adds the following procedures:

> AUTOREGR, BMDP, CLUSTER, CONTENTS, CONVERT,
> DELETE, GLM, HISTOGRAM, MATRIX, NEIGHBOR, NLIN,
> PROBIT, SAS 72, SCATTER, SCORE, SPECTRA, STANDARD,
> SYSREG, TTEST and VARCOMP.

Some of these are concerned with the more flexible input, internal manipulation, and display of data (CONTENTS, DE-LETE, HISTOGRAM). Some enable the user to access other packages via SAS 76 (BMDP, SAS 72) or to convert data sets generated by other packages (SAS 72, SPSS, OSIRIS, BMDP, DATA TEXT) to SAS 76 format using the procedure CONVERT. The remainder represent the addition of new statistical programs in various areas (time series—AUTOREGR, SPECTRA; clustering techniques—CLUSTER, NEIGHBOR; special regressions—NLIN, SYSREG) and the addition of sub-packages. Thus GLM is a master program for the general linear model which can be used for all balanced analysis of variance situations and for linear regressions of any order, and MATRIX is a valuable set of programs for creating and handling matrices and for matrix operations. A general-purpose table builder is soon to be added and will round off this very valuable statistical package.

LITERATURE CITED

Bailey, N. T. J. 1957. The Mathematical Theory of Epidemics. Charles Griffin & Co. Ltd., London.

Barr, A. J., J. H. Goodnight, and J. Service. 1972. A User's Guide to the Statistical Analysis System. Student Supply Stores, North Carolina State University, Raleigh, N.C.

Barr, A. J., J. H. Goodnight, J. P. Sall, et al. 1976. A User's Guide to SAS 76. SAS Institute Inc. Sparks Press, Raleigh, N.C.

Dixon, W. J. (ed.) 1975. Biomedical Computer Program. Health Sciences Computing Facility/U.C.L.A. University of California Press, Berkely, 1975.

Feurzeig, W, P. Munter, J. Swets, and M. Breen. 1964. Computer-aided Teaching in Medical Diagnosis. J. Med. Educ. 39:746–754.

Glaser, J. H. 1971. Health-Information Systems: A Crisis or Just More of the Usual. Amer. J. Pub. Health 61(8):1524.

Kilpatrick, S. J. 1971. An Alternative to the Standardized Score in Grading a Multiple Choice Examination. J. Exp. Educ. 39(4):61.

Krieg, A. F., J. J. Johnson, Jr., C. McDonald, E. Cotlove. 1971. Clinical Laboratory Computerization. University Park Press, Baltimore.

Ledley, R. S. 1967. Computer Aids to Clinical Treatment Evaluation. Oper. Res. 15(4):694–705.

Mainland, D. 1968. How Much Computerized Nonsense from Hospital Records, p. 23–28. In D. Mainland, Notes on Biometry in Medical Research. Veterans Administration, Suppl. 4., Washington, D.C.

Nie, N. H., C. H. Hull, J. G. Jenkins, E. T. 1975. Statistical Package for the Social Sciences. 2nd Ed. McGraw-Hill Book Company, New York.

Westlake, G. E., and J. L. Bennington. 1972. Automation and Management in the Clinical Laboratory. University Park Press, Baltimore.

Wilson, P. D. 1970. Smoothing and Prediction of a Multivariate Non-stationary Time Series. Presented at Southern Region Educational Board Summer Research Conference in Statistics, Mountain Lake, Virginia.

FURTHER READING

Brandt, E. N., Jr. 1966a. The Future Effect of the Computer and the Research Scientist on Medical Practice. Medical College of Virginia Quarterly 2(4):234.

Brandt, E. N., Jr. 1966b. Applications of Computers to Medicine. Medical College of Virginia Quarterly 2(4):238.

Ledley, R. S. 1965. Use of Computers in Biology and Medicine. McGraw-Hill Book Company, New York.

Lusted, L. B. 1968. Introduction to Medical Decision Making. Charles C Thomas, Springfield, Ill.

Lusted, L. G., and R. W. Coffin. 1967. Prime—An Automated Information System for Hospitals and Biomedical Research Laboratories. Year Book Medical Publishers, Chicago.

Rustagi, J. S. 1968. Dynamic Programming Model of Patient Care. Math. Biosc. 3:141.

Wilson, V. E., and A. B. Lindberg. 1965. Laboratory Data Handling System is Automatic. Hosp. Manag. 99:84.

13

Design of Investigation

13.1 INTRODUCTION

In Chapter 4 the theory and some of the concepts of epidemiological studies and sample surveys were introduced. Here an overview of these research studies is given from the statistical viewpoint. The importance of selecting a sample at random from a well-defined population has been stressed in Chapter 4 and elsewhere. We shall see by reference to the literature that it is often not possible to take random samples. The conclusions of those papers in which a nonrandom sample is used are interpreted as though the samples were random. Thus, the postulated effects or relationships described in the references quoted below (when based on a nonrandom sample) might be due to biases introduced by the method of selection. This dichotomy between the population of interest and the sample studied is apparent in various types of investigation. Studies can be described statistically as descriptive, comparative, experimental, mixed (comparative and experimental), and as other nonexperimental investigations.

13.2 DESCRIPTIVE INVESTIGATIONS

Enumeration of the total population and collection of information of interest provide a valid statistical description of the population. The reader will be familiar with the population census and with hospital and other types of census. Stevenson and Cheeseman (1956) claim to have detected all cases of deaf mutism in

253

Northern Ireland. This is an example of a census or complete ascertainment of all individuals with a given characteristic in a well-defined population. It is, however, often wasteful to enumerate the whole population when less than absolute accuracy is required. This is the reason for taking a sample survey in which a small fraction of the population is studied so that estimates for the total population can be made. Since sampling introduces variation in the resultant estimates, statistical techniques are used to describe realistic limits for the size of this variation (Chapters 7, 8, 9). Sample data may be examined to discover the relationships among variables and to suggest the underlying mechanisms of the system. It is generally assumed that a relationship found between two variables in a sample will also be found between these variables in the population. The best way of validating this assumption is to draw a second sample, independent of the first, and examine the data to see whether the same relationship holds. This is the approach used in regression and **discriminant analysis**. Thus, Rittenbury et al. (1965) developed, by means of discriminant analysis, a formula to predict the prognosis for future burn patients from the survival characteristics of past burn patients.

13.3 COMPARATIVE INVESTIGATIONS

Almost all studies are comparative in one way or another. Comparisons are made between the results from two sets of data, or the results from a set of data may be compared with historical results or with the expectation or belief of a knowledgeable person. Thus, the statement that 35% of all drivers involved in automobile accidents had been drinking is really a comparison of this percentage with the percentage of all drivers who had been drinking. Two populations can, of course, be compared without recourse to statistical inference (e.g., Americans have a higher average per capita income than Russians). Two samples can be compared to test whether they come from the same or different populations (see Section 9.5). Thus, the belief that men are genetically XY and women XX is based on chromosome studies of tissue samples from some men and women. Clearly, we cannot test all mankind. Note, however, that as more information became available and more precise techniques were evolved the original genetic classification of the sexes had to be expanded to allow for other combinations of the X and Y chromosomes, e.g., XXY (Jacobs, Price, and Law, 1970). In contrast to experimental investigations, nothing is done to alter the individual items studied. Therefore, the observed differences between the samples can be imputed to be real differences in the characteristics of the populations (after random sampling variation has been ruled out).

Occasionally, it is useful to describe a population superficially and to draw a sample in order to gather additional information—to study relationships among the variables, etc. This naturally leads to a comparison of the characteristics of the sample with the known characteristics of the population in order to check that the sample is representative. Richardson (1964) uses this approach in an epidemiological study of prostatic hyperplasia and social class.

13.4 EXPERIMENTAL INVESTIGATIONS

In an experiment, the investigator deliberately intervenes, i.e., he changes some items and then tries to measure the effect of these changes. This intervention is usually called a **treatment** of the material, but a treatment can mean anything deliberately imposed by the investigator. Individual items that receive no treatment are generally called **controls**.

As in comparative investigations, the experimenter can "treat" the whole population or he can "treat" a sample of the population and use preconceived ideas or historical evidence to deduce whether the treatment affected the population in the observed response variables. Hill (1952) showed the dangers in this and recommended that "controlled clinical trials" be used instead. A **controlled clinical trial** is one in which a sample of suitable subjects is selected and is randomly divided into "treatment" and "control" groups. The argument is that, apart from random influences in the allocation of individuals to one group or another, the only way that the groups differ is that one group is treated and the other one is not. Significant differences in the reactions or responses of the two groups can then be attributed to treatment or lack of treatment. In medical investigations, both doctors and patients should remain in ignorance of who is on treatment and who is not. This is to prevent biases in the patient's response or in the physician's evaluation of these responses. These clinical trials are called **double blind** in that neither the subject nor the person recording the subject's responses knows which group the subject is in. The control group in a double-blind clinical trial receives a neutral or ineffective treatment in a manner identical to that used in the treatment group. Thus, in a double-blind clinical trial of ampicillin for typhoid (Russell, Sutherland, and Walker, 1966), identical capsules of ampicillin and an inert substance were given orally to patients in the treatment and **placebo** (or control) group, respectively. The design of experiments goes far beyond these elementary considerations of clinical trials in which only one treatment is considered.

Factorial experiments are those in which the simultaneous effects of several treatments at different levels are estimated. The first objective of a good factorial design is to provide estimates of important effects that are separable from other effects or influ-

Table 13.1. Number of women on given diet and level of fluid intake

	Diet		
Fluid intake	A	B	C
Minimal	3	3	3
Moderate	3	3	3
Excess	3	3	3

Table 13.2. Number of women on given diet and level of fluid intake

	Diet		
Fluid intake	A	B	C
Minimal	9		
Moderate		9	
Excess			9

Table 13.3. Number of women on given diet with excess fluid intake

Diet	A	B	C
Excess Fluids	9	9	9

Table 13.4. Number of women on diet B at different levels of fluid intake

Fluid intake	Diet B
Minimal	9
Moderate	9
Excess	9

ences. In general, in a balanced design, one can estimate the effects of a factor averaged over different levels of other factors.

Example. In a hypothetical experiment to determine the effect of different diets, A, B, and C, and the effect the amount of fluid intake can have on weight changes in women, two different experimental strategies might be followed, as in Tables 13.1 and 13.2, where the numbers indicate the number of women allocated to different treatment modalities of diet and fluid intake. Of course, the research worker might not do the experiment either of these ways. He might use the single-factor design shown in Table 13.3 to find which diet (say B) has the greatest effect on weight when there is no limitation on fluid intake and then repeat the experiment using diets with different amounts of fluid intake (Table 13.4). The above procedure implies that he is interested in the combination of diet and fluid intake that most decreases body weight. If this is so, then the "one factor at a time" approach is inefficient (more people, more time) and may even be misleading because of **interaction** (diet C with moderate fluid intake may give best results). Many efficient experimental designs are now available for use in medical research.

13.5 MIXED INVESTIGATIONS

Mixed investigations are combinations of comparative investigations and experimental investigations. In studies of samples from different populations, the differences (if real) are ascribed to differences among the populations. In experimental studies, care is taken to choose a sample from only one population, and the population is then divided randomly into different groups, so that differences can be ascribed to treatments. A mixed investigation is one in which samples are taken from different populations and different treatments are imposed on the samples. Real differences among the samples are then due either to differences among the populations or to differences in the effects of the treatments or conceivably to synergistic effects between the treatments and members of the different populations. When it is not possible to say which source caused the response, the investigation is said to be **confounded**! Very often, however, confounding cannot be avoided.

Example.   In a three-year study of the effects of influenza vaccine on absenteeism in a factory (Richardson and Kilpatrick, 1964), it was considered inadvisable to randomize the vaccine. Instead, in each of the three years each employee decided whether he wanted to be treated with the vaccine that year. Since those who chose vaccination were likely to be different from those who chose not to be vaccinated (with respect to their susceptibility to influenza, etc.), it was not possible to separate the effects of vaccination from the characterics of the volunteers. Fortunately, no significant differences were found to exist between the frequency of absence caused by sickness in vaccinated and nonvaccinated individuals!

Another common type of confounding is when different treatments are combined. Thus, in Table 13.2, diets and fluid intake are confounded since each diet is associated with only one level of fluid intake instead of with all three levels. It is therefore impossible to tell whether the diet or the amount of fluid was important in this weight-loss investigation.

13.6   OTHER TYPES OF INVESTIGATIONS

In practice, it is often impossible to experiment because this would adversely affect the system and the investigator's relationships with it. Thus, no surgeon would agree to discharge his patients, chosen at random, at fixed intervals after a given operation to investigate the optimal number of hospital days in recovery. Even though such an experiment might unequivocally answer questions regarding postoperative care, his position would be that his concern is to provide the best care to each individual patient. In such situations, recourse is made to mathematical modeling or simulation, in which the major determinants of the system are related functionally. As in the case of statistical analyses, the model could be tested by comparing its predictions against real data, which had not been used to create the model. When he is confident that his mathematical model is robust, i.e., that it will describe the system under various conditions, the investigator can begin experimenting on the model—making deliberate changes in the levels of the determinant factors and observing the results of these *in the model.* In this way, he can find a theoretically optimal arrangement of this system. His next task is to convince the administrator, surgeon, or other person in charge of the system he studied that his results are beneficial, if not optimal, *in practice.* Note that, in this context, Forrester (1962) and others claim that decision makers cannot really comprehend the long-term results of policy changes in complex situations with more than six inter-acting factors, and that recourse to a computer model is essential to predict the outcome of decisions in these circumstances.

The operations analyst has the same goals as the systems modeler except that he typically studies components of the sys-tem rather than the total system. His reason for doing so is that he is interested in practical solutions. A body of techniques has developed in operations analysis or operations research concerning the allocation of scarce resources, scheduling, queueing, inventory control, etc., and many texts have been published describing these techniques (see below).

13.7 PLANNING AND CRITIQUE

The reader should now be prepared to apply the ideas presented here. There are two usual ways of doing so. One is to plan and carry through your own investigation, and the second is to use this background to evaluate what others have done and reported in the literature. A consultant statistician is experienced at translating his knowledge into action both in planning investigations and in evaluating the work of others. He will not, however, know as much of the field of application as you will and so each of you will complement the other.

Authors of statistical texts are loath to set down the principles by which statisticians translate their theoretical knowledge into action. This is because it is difficult to cover all situations with a set of rules or guidelines. Mainland (1964) lists a series of questions that indicate the procedures to be followed in any investigation. These questions are grouped into ten different areas covering:

1. The nature of the research and the attitudes of the researchers
2. Purpose and general method of investigation
3. The population and sample
4. Subdivision of population and sample
5. Skeleton layout for results
6. Interpretation after an experiment
7. Interpretation after a survey
8. Sample size
9. Collection, recording and examination of the data
10. Lost information

The evaluation of a research report on paper can similarly be made in terms of Mainland's questions. More specifically, Colton (1974) gives an outline for a critique of a report developed by Rutstein, which is reproduced below:

OUTLINE FOR CRITIQUE OF A MEDICAL REPORT

I. Object or hypothesis
   A. What are the objectives of the study or the questions to be answered?
   B. What is the population to which the investigators intend to refer their findings?

II. Design of the investigation
   A. Was the study an experiment, planned observations, or an analysis of records?
   B. How was the sample selected? Are there possible sources of selection which would make the sample atypical or nonrepresentative? If so, what provision was made to deal with this bias?
   C. What is the nature of the control group or standard of comparison?

III. Observations
A. Are there clear definitions of the terms used, including diagnostic criteria, measurements made, and criteria of outcome?
B. Was the method of classification or of measurement consistent for all the subjects and relevant to the objectives of the investigation? Are there possible biases in measurement and, if so, what provisions were made to deal with them?
C. Are the observations reliable and reproducible?

IV. Presentation of findings
A. Are the findings presented clearly, objectively, and in sufficient detail to enable the reader to judge them for himself?
B. Are the findings internally consistent, i.e., do the numbers add up properly, can the different tables be reconciled, etc.?

V. Analysis
A. Are the data worthy of statistical analysis? If so, are the methods of statistical analysis appropriate to the source and nature of the data and is the analysis correctly performed and interpreted?
B. Is there sufficient analysis to determine whether "significant differences" may in fact be due to lack of comparability of the groups in sex or age distribution, in clinical characteristics, or in other relevant variables?

VI. Conclusions
Which conclusions are justified by the findings? Which are not? Are the conclusions relevant to the questions posed by the investigators?

Both Mainland (1964) and Colton (1974) may be consulted for further details on the planning and critique of health care investigations. However, there is no substitute for experience. Most users of statistics learn by applying common statistical techniques to a series of real-life situations and referring to tests and/or experts as needed. It is hoped that this book will help in the interpretation of health care information and will lead its readers to independent research.

LITERATURE CITED

Cochran, W. G. 1965. The Planning of Observational Studies of Human Populations. J. Roy. Statist. Soc. Ser. A 128:234.
Colton, T. 1974. Statistics in Medicine. Little, Brown & Co., Boston.
Forrester, J. W. 1962. Managerial Decision Making, pp. 37–67. In Green-

berger, M. (Ed.). Computers and the World of the Future. MIT Press, Cambridge.

Hill, A. B. 1952. The Clinical Trial. New Engl. J. Med. 247:113.

Jacobs, P. A., W. H. Price, and P. Law, (Ed.). 1970. Human Population Cytogenetics. The Williams & Wilkins Company, Baltimore.

Mainland, D. 1964. Elementary Medical Statistics. 2nd Ed. W. B. Saunders Company, Philadelphia.

Richardson, I. M. 1964. Prostatic Hyperplasia and Social Class. Brit. J. Prev. Soc. Med. 18(3):157.

Richardson, I. M., and S. J. Kilpatrick. 1964. Influenza Immunization. A Three-Year Study in a Factory Population. Med. Off. 3:5.

Rittenbury, M. S., et al. 1965. Factors Significantly Affecting Mortality in the Burned Patient. J. Trauma 5(5):587.

Russell, E. M., A. Sutherland and W. Walker. 1966. Ampicillin for Persistent Typhoid Excreters Including a Clinical Trial in Convalescence. Brit. Med. J. 2:555.

Stevenson, A. C., and E. A. Cheeseman. 1965. Hereditary Deaf Mutism with Particular References to Northern Ireland. Ann. Hum. Genet. 20(3): 177–231.

FURTHER READING

Blalock, H. M. 1961. Causal Inferences in Non-experimental Research. University of North Carolina, Chapel Hill.

Campbell, D. T., and J. C. Stanley. 1966. Experimental and Quasi-experimental Designs for Research. Rand McNally & Company, Chicago.

Cox, D. R. 1958. Planning of Experiments. John Wiley & Sons Inc., New York.

Churchman, C. W., R. L. Ackoff, and E. L. Arnoff. 1957. Introduction to Operations Research. John Wiley & Sons Inc., New York.

Fisher, R. A. 1960. The Design of Experiments. 7th Ed. Oliver & Boyd Ltd., Edinburgh.

Flagle, C. D., W. H. Huggins, and R. H. Roy. 1960. Operations Research and System Engineering. The Johns Hopkins University Press, Baltimore.

Hill, A. B. (Ed.). 1960. Controlled Clinical Trials. Blackwell Scientific Publications Ltd., Oxford.

Kilpatrick, S. J. 1969. The Role of Operations Research in a University Hospital—A Review and Bibliography. MCV/Q 5(2):61.

Mainland, D. 1964. Elementary Medical Statistics. 2nd Ed. W. B. Saunders Company, Philadelphia.

Wilson, E. B. 1952. An Introduction to Scientific Research. McGraw-Hill Book Company, New York.

Appendix

Mathematical Expressions

#	number of
$\sqrt{}$	square root
=	equals sign
$\approx$	approximately equal
>	greater than
$\geq$	greater than or equal to
<	less than
$\leq$	less than or equal to
| |	absolute value, i.e., $|{-3}| = 3$
3!	three factorial, or $3 \times 2 \times 1$

$\dbinom{5}{3}$ the number of ways 3 things can be chosen from 5 things, or

$$\frac{5!}{3!\,2!} = 10$$

∞	infinity
$\sum$	sum of, e.g., $\sum\limits_{i=1}^{3} x_i = x_1 + x_2 + x_3$
$\therefore$	therefore
$\rightarrow$	estimates

Notation

a the intercept, an estimate of α

b the regression coefficient, the slope of the regression, an estimate of β

c a constant

d a constant

D_t a smoothed time series

E expected number in the cell of a table, calculated as the product of the row and column totals divided by the grand total

e the error term in a regression equation

$\mathcal{E}$ expected value

$\mathcal{E}(\bar{x})$ expected value of the sample mean, i.e., the mean of means from repeated random samples of fixed size

$\mathcal{E}(p)$ expected value of the sample proportion, i.e., the mean of proportions from repeated random samples of fixed size

f a fraction or a frequency

f_x the frequency with which x occurs

f_i the frequency with which x_i occurs

F Fisher's statistic or $(s')^2/(s'')^2$ where $s' \geqslant s''$

i a counter by which measures are identified (see $x_i, x_{(i)}$)

k a constant

m the number in a sample of size n with a given attribute

N the size of the population

n the size of the sample

n' the size of the first sample

n'' the size of the second sample

O the observed number in the cell of a table

p a sample proportion, i.e., $p = m/n$

p_l the lower confidence limit of $\mathcal{P}$

p_u the upper confidence limit of $\mathcal{P}$

$\mathcal{P}$ the proportion in the population with the given attribute; hence, also, the probability that an item selected at random from the population will have the attribute

P probability

$P(A)$ the probability that A occurs

$P(AB)$ the probability that A and B occur

$P(A \mid B)$ the probability that A occurs given that B has occurred; i.e., $P(p \mid n, \mathcal{P})$ means the probability that a sample proportion occurs in a sample size n from a population $\mathcal{P}\%$ of which has the attribute

Q the proportion in the population not having the attribute, i.e., $Q = 1 - \mathcal{P}$

r the correlation coefficient between pairs of measures in a sample

R^2 the multiple correlation coefficient

R_t a trend in a time series

s	the sample standard deviation of a measure
s'	the standard deviation in the first of two samples
s''	the standard deviation in the second of two samples
s_x	the sample standard deviation of x
$s_{\bar{x}}$	the estimated standard error of $\bar{x}$
s_p	the estimated standard error of p
s_t	a seasonal effect in a time series
t	t test statistic, occurring in the text in different forms; a variable representing time
w	the sample range; a weighting factor
x	the symbol used for a measure, a predictor variable
x_i	the ith value occurring in the sample or population
$x_{(i)}$	the ith value occurring in the sample after the observations have been ranked in increasing order
$\bar{x}$	the sample mean
$\bar{x}'$	the sample mean in the first of two samples
$\bar{x}''$	the sample mean in the second of two samples (in general, "prime" and "double prime" are used to identify the first and second of two samples, respectively)
$\bar{x}_{50}$	the sample median
$\bar{x}_o$	the sample mode
y	a response or dependent measure
y_t	the value of y at time t
$\hat{y}$	a predicted value for y
z	the standard normal deviate
α	the "true" intercept, the value in the population estimated by a
β	the "true" regression coefficient, the value in the population estimated by b
λ	the substitution constant
μ	the population mean
μ_{50}	the population median
μ_o	the population mode
ν	degrees of freedom
ρ	the correlation coefficient in a population
σ	the population standard deviation
σ_x	the population standard deviation of a measure x
$\sigma_{\bar{x}}$	the population standard error of the sample mean $\bar{x}$
σ_p	the population standard error of the sample proportion p

σ^2 the population variance

χ^2 the chi-squared statistic

♂   male

♀   female

γ a weighting factor between 0 and 1 used in exponential smoothing

Definition of Terms

ACCEPTANCE SAMPLING—a branch of sampling in which, on the basis of a small sample of a consignment, the decision is made to accept or reject the whole consignment.

ACCURACY—the difference between a sample estimate and the population value that is estimated. Accuracy is thought of as having two components, sampling variation and non-sampling error.

AGGREGATIVE FALLACY—the often fallacious assumption that a relationship between variables of aggregates will also hold between elements in the population. *Example*: If a direct relationship is shown between average age of patient and average length of stay among a sample of hospitals, it does not follow that the same relationship will hold between the age and length of hospital stay of individual patients in the sample.

ANALYTICAL SURVEY—a survey whose primary purpose is to compare sub-groups of the population sampled.

BAR GRAPH—a graph of a frequency table in which the measurement or classification is given along one axis and where the frequencies are represented by columns with lengths proportional to the frequencies observed.

BIAS—describes a systematic error in a sample estimate: the difference between the value being estimated and the expected value of the sample estimate. *Example*: The standard deviation calculated from a sample is a biased estimate of the population standard deviation.

BINOMIAL DISTRIBUTION—If a random sample of n units are taken from a population in which $\mathcal{P}$ of the units have a given attribute $(0 < \mathcal{P} < 1)$, then the probability that m in the sample have the attribute $(0 \leqslant m \leqslant n)$ is given by $P(m/n, \mathcal{P}) = \binom{n}{m} \mathcal{P}^m (1 - \mathcal{P})^{n-m}$.

CENSUS—the examination or measurement of each member of a population—a sampling fraction of 100%.

CHANCE POINT—a branch in a decision tree at which one of several events must happen by chance (or at any rate, outside the control of the decision maker).

CLASSIFICATION—a grouping of items according to the level of a common attribute into a number of mutually exclusive and exhaustive classes. (In some instances, a classification may be based on a grouped measurement. *Example*: Classifying anyone over six feet as tall).

COMPONENT PARTS GRAPH—a graph in which a given shape (usually a rectangle or circle) is divided into parts with areas proportional to the amount of the various components of a system.

CONDITIONAL PROBABILITY—if the probability that an event A occurs is dependent on whether or not a prior event B has occurred, then we say the probability of A is conditional on B and write $P(A/B)$ to mean the (conditional) probability of A given that B has occurred. Consequently $P(A$ and $B) = P(B) \cdot P(A/B)$.

CONFIDENCE LIMITS—two values within which a population parameter is said to lie with a specified probability (or confidence).

CONFOUNDED—the situation (frequently occurring) in which the effects produced by different treatments cannot be separated.

CONTROL—a group of items that are untreated in order to provide an appropriate comparison for the treated group or groups.

CONTROL CHART—a graph showing the results of small-scale repeated sampling of an ongoing process. It generally consists of two lines between which the sample average must fall. A sample average falling outside these lines is interpreted to mean that the process has gone or is going out of control, i.e., that nonrandom influences are at work.

CONTROLLED CLINICAL TRIAL—an experiment with a treated and a control group (also known as a clinical trial).

CORRELATION COEFFICIENT—a measure of the positive or negative association between two variates, generally two measures or two ranks.

COST FUNCTION—a formula relating the cost of a procedure to its several components.

COUNT—the number of items falling into a certain class (a classification is thus a count in a number of mutually exclusive and exhaustive classes).

CRITICAL VALUE—the tabulated value of the test statistic that corresponds to a specified probability or level of significance.

CYCLE—fluctuations around the trend line, often of variable duration.

DECISION POINT—a branch in a decision tree at which a choice has to be made about which of several decisions to adopt.

DECISION TREE—a graphical representation of a complex decision process, showing the alternative choices and the expected outcome and consequences.

DEGREES OF FREEDOM—loosely, the number of independent components in a test statistic. Thus, in some cases, the number of independent values minus the number of independent constraints placed upon them. The definition varies from application to application.

DIGITAL COMPUTER—a machine that compares, adds, substracts, etc., on the basis of discrete electromagnetic pulses that represent the numbers 0 and 1 (or some other set of integers).

DISCRIMINANT ANALYSIS—a multi-variable statistical procedure by which items may be allocated to one of several populations on the basis of a function derived from the characteristics of several populations.

DOUBLE BLIND—neither the individuals receiving the treatment nor the persons evaluating the outcome knowing who got what. (A **placebo** is often given to the control group.)

DOUBLED—TAILED TESTS—a significance test in which either a positive or a significant difference may occur. Also called a two-tailed test.

EPIDEMIOLOGY—the study of the natural occurrence of disease and its causes. The word 'epidemiology' is no longer restricted to the study of infectious diseases. *Example*: The epidemiology of mental health.

EXCEPTION REPORTING—the procedure by which only anomalous information is provided to a decision-maker.

EXPECTED; EXPECTATION; EXPECTED VALUE—the expectation (or expected value) of a sample statistic is the mean of all values of the statistic produced by repeated random sampling.

EXPONENTIAL SMOOTHING—an average of the current and all previous values of a time series, with weights decreasing geometrically from the present to the past.

FACTORIAL EXPERIMENT—an experiment in which several treatments are evaluated simultaneously and in which each combination of treatment levels is represented.

FLOW CHART—a symbolic representation of the processes occurring in any activity, showing the temporal interconnections of component activities.

FRAME—an enumeration or listing of the population to be sampled.

FREQUENCY DISTRIBUTION—a specification of the way in which the frequencies of members of a population are distributed according to the variable of interest. The frequency distribution is often given in the form of a frequency table.

FREQUENCY TABLE—a grouping of a series of observations, showing the count or frequency of observations falling into successive groups or classes.

HISTOGRAM—a graphical representation of a frequency table with frequencies represented by vertical columns proportional in area to the observed frequencies. Hence, histograms generally show the variate of interest in equal intervals along the horizontal axis.

INDEPENDENT—two variables are independent if the joint probability of the two variables is the product of the individual probabilities. Hence, the joint frequency of any values of the two variables is the product of their separate frequencies.

INDEX—a composite number combining two or more different variables in a single figure.

INFANT MORTALITY RATE—the number of deaths of liveborn children under one year of age registered in a given year divided by the number of live births registered in that year. I.M.R. = 20 per 1000, approximately.

INTERACTION—a measure of the extent to which the effect on the response variate of changing the level of one factor depends on the level of another factor.

INVERSE SAMPLING—random sampling in which items are selected until those with a given characteristic reach a specified number.

MEAN—the arithmetic average.

MEASUREMENT—a continuous quantity based on a scale with a fixed but divisible unit.

MEASUREMENT UNITS—components of a sampling unit that are examined when the sampling unit is selected. *Example:* If a household were selected as a sampling unit, then, possibly, each member of that household might be examined (measurement units). Often the sampling unit and the measurement unit are synonymous. *Example*: The average length of stay of patients in a hospital might be estimated by taking a sample of beds (sampling units) and listing the length of stay of the last patient who occupied that bed.

MEDIAN—the middle value of a series of values arranged in order of size. When the number of values being averaged is even, the median is the mean of the middle pair of values.

MODE—the most frequently occurring value in a series of values.

MORBIDITY RATE—the number of illnesses experienced or reported by a given population in a given period divided by the mid-period population at risk.

MOVING AVERAGE—a weighted average of adjoining values in a time series, which, when repeatedly applied over the whole time series, removes excessive variation, i.e., which "smooths" the series.

NOMOGRAM—a figure to facilitate numerical calculations or conversions. Scales of different variables are drawn on straight lines or curves in such a way that corresponding values lie on an intersecting straight line.

NORMAL DISTRIBUTION—If $f(x)$, the frequency with which a given value x occurs in a population is related to the mean (μ) and the standard deviation (σ) by:

$$f(x) = \frac{1}{\sigma\sqrt{2\pi}}\exp\left\{-1/2\left(\frac{x-\mu}{\sigma}\right)^2\right\}$$

then x follows a normal distribution.

NORMAL RANGE; NORMAL LIMITS—the range or limits outside which all abnormal individuals are assumed to fall.

ODDS—the ratio of the probability of an event to the complementary probability of the non-event. *Example*: If the probability that a newborn is a boy is 0.51, then boy/girl odds at birth are 51:49.

OUTLIER—a value that is so different from other members of the sample that it is suspected to belong to a different population.

PARENT DISTRIBUTION—sometimes known as the underlying distribution: the parent distribution is the distribution of the original observation in the total population.

PLACEBO—an inert treatment undetectable in its methods of administration (and side effects) from the treatments under investigation.

PICTOGRAPH—a figure in which the number of times a symbol is repeated represents the frequency with which that value or characteristic occurs.

PILOT SURVEY—a small-scale survey (cheap and convenient) conducted before the main survey to provide information for the subsequent design of the main survey, both in improving the survey instruments and in the selection of the sample.

POLYNOMIAL—a form with two or more terms but used here in the sense of a form composed of a variable and its powers. *Example*: $a + bx + cx^2$.

POPULATION—the total group or body of items or individuals of interest.

PROBABILITY—a value ranging from zero (an impossible event) to one (a certain event) that describes the "chance" that an event will occur. Probability concepts may be derived either from "degrees of belief" or from frequency arguments about idealized events.

PROBABILITY SAMPLING—sampling in which each item in the population has a specified probability of selection.

QUARTILES—three values of a variate that divide a frequency distribution into four equal parts, the median being the middle quartile.

RANDOM SAMPLING—a procedure by which each potential sample in the population has a predetermined probability of selection.

RATE—the number of events occurring in a population in a given period divided by the mid-term population—usually expressed as per 1000. Some rates however do not follow this definition. *Example*: See **Infant Mortality Rate**.

REGRESSION; REGRESSION COEFFICIENT—the name of a statistical procedure by which a straight line or curve is fitted (generally by least squares) to repeated groups of variables, one of which, the response variable, is thought to depend on the others. The regression coefficient is, in general, the coefficient of any term in the resulting relationship. In linear regression, where a straight line is fitted to pairs of observations, it is the slope of this regression line.

RELATIVE FREQUENCY—the absolute frequency (or count of the number of observations that fall in a certain interval or class) divided by the total number of observations—also expressed as a percentage.

ROBUSTNESS—a statistical procedure is said to be robust if it is insensitive to the underlying assumptions, i.e., large departures from the original assumptions are required before the results of the procedure become misleading.

SAMPLE—a subgroup of a population, generally selected in order to provide information about the population from which it was drawn.

SAMPLE SURVEY—the selection and examination of a fraction of a population in order to estimate the characteristics of the population (but see also **Analytical Survey**).

SAMPLING DISTRIBUTION—an estimate of a population parameter will vary from sample to sample. Sample estimates will, therefore, be distributed around their mean. The distribution of estimates from all possible random samples of a given size is known as the sampling distribution of the estimate.

SAMPLING FRACTION—the proportion of the sampling units in the population that constitute the sample.

SAMPLING UNITS—for the purposes of sampling, the population is considered to be divided into sampling units, i.e., discrete distinguishable items. *Example*: In terms of a human population, city blocks and households might be the sampling unit in different surveys.

SAMPLING VARIATION—the differences among estimates derived from repeated samples of the same size.

SEASONAL EFFECT—deviations from the trend line that recur at certain times, i.e., a cycle of fixed period generally not longer than a year.

SENSITIVITY ANALYSIS—a critique of a forecasting technique as applied to a given situation. The analyst uses ancillary information, often non-quantified, to judge how far he can extrapolate or to improve forecasts.

SERIAL CORRELATION—the correlation between observations in a time series that are one, two or more apart.

SIGNIFICANCE—statistically, a significant effect is one that is unlikely to be due solely to chance. A statistically significant effect, therefore, is one thought to be real, even though the effect itself might be unimportant.

SINGLE-TAILED TEST—a significance test in which only a significant difference is of interest in one direction (either positive or negative). Also called a one-tailed test.

SPECTRAL ANALYSIS—a technique that decomposes a continuous time series into its principal periodic frequencies.

STANDARD DEVIATION—the square root of the variance of a population or sample of measurements. The standard deviation is in the same units as the original measurements and describes the scatter or dispersion of either the parent distribution or the frequency distribution of the original observations in the sample.

STANDARD ERROR—the square root of the variance of a sample statistic.

The standard error measures the scatter or dispersion of the sampling distribution of this statistic.

STATISTIC—originally an item of (numerical) information on a member of a population. More often it is used in "statistics" to mean a value which summarizes the information in a sample. Technically, therefore, a statistic is a function of the values of a sample.

STATISTICAL MAP—a map of a geographical region on which statistical information is superimposed.

STATISTICS—plural of **statistic**—more often, the name given to the discipline concerned with the collection, analysis, and interpretation of experiments, surveys, and observational studies.

STRATIFYING—instead of taking a sample from a population, the population may first be divided into sub-populations (strata) and a sample taken from each strata. If the relative size of each stratum is known and strata tend to group similar sampling units (with respect to the variable of interest, the precision of the overall estimate will be improved).

SUBSTITUTION CONSTANT—a numerical value establishing the equivalence between the units of two different scales.

SURVEY INSTRUMENT—generally a questionnaire or other fixed procedure to obtain the desired information from sampled individuals.

SYSTEMATIC SAMPLING—nonrandom sampling in which every k^{th} item is selected, often after a randomly selected start.

TEST STATISTIC—a statistic specifically calculated to test a statistical hypothesis.

TIME SERIES—a set of sequential observations in time that generally show a serial correlation. Many time series are based on observations made a constant interval apart.

TOLERANCE LIMITS—two values within which a specified proportion of the population is said to lie with a given probability.

TREATMENT—any deliberate manipulation of items in an experiment.

TREND—a systematic increase or decrease in a variable over time.

TURNING POINT—in a continuous time series, a local maximum or minimum. In a discrete time series, each value that lies outside the range of its two neighbors is a turning point.

UTILITY—subjective value measured in terms of an equivalent expected gain of money.

UNBIASED ESTIMATOR—when the expectation of a sample estimate equals the population parameter estimated, the estimate is said to be unbiased.

VARIANCE—the second moment of a frequency distribution about its mean—the mean squared deviation. The variance σ^2 of the parent distribution is estimated unbiasedly by s^2 in a random sample of observations.

VITAL STATISTICS—demography—the description of a human population in terms of its vital events (births, marriages, deaths).

WEIGHT—a numerical coefficient that measures the subjective importance, frequency, or information of different outcomes or observations relative to the complete set.

Answers to Exercises

CHAPTER 2

2.1 Measure = M; Classification = C; Table 2.2 (M); Figure 2.3 (C); Figure 2.6 (C); Figure 2.8 (C); Figure 2.9 (C); Figure 2.10 (C); Figure 2.12 ($M,M,C,C,$); Table 2.3 (C,C); Figure 2.13 (M).

2.2 C = count, $\bar{C}$ = not a count; Table 2.1 (C); Figure 2.13 (C); Figure 2.2 ($\bar{C}$); Figure 3.1 ($C,\bar{C}$); Figure 2.17 ($\bar{C}$).

2.3 Absolute frequencies in Table 2.4 calculated by multiplying percentages in each row of the table by the total number of facilities given for that row in Table 2.5. We cannot do this for residents and employees without tables like Table 2.4 showing the percentage distribution of residents and employees.

2.5 a) 27
 b) 40

2.6 From 17 to 20.

2.7 As a 6 $\times$ 1 frequency table enumerating the number of tumors (classified as benign parotid, malignant parotid, benign submaxillary, malignant submaxillary, benign sublingual, malignant sublingual). The seven tables are:

	Benign	Malignant	Total
Parotid	501	231	732
Submaxillary	47	54	101
Sublingual	0	3	3
Salivary	548	288	836

	Parotid	Submaxillary	Sublingual	Total
Benign	501	47	0	548
Malignant	231	54	3	288
Neoplasms	732	101	3	836

Either the two 3 $\times$ 1 independent tables or the three independent 2 $\times$ 1 tables.

2.8 Counts; a one-way frequency table.

2.9 a)

	Nurse 1			Nurse 2			
	Day	Night	Total	Day	Night	Total	Total
Wt. loss	1	5	6	5	3	8	14
No wt. loss	6	2	8	1	5	6	14
Total	7	7	14	6	8	14	28

b) 8/15 or 53%

c) Nurse 1: 5/7 or 71%, Nurse 2: 3/8 or 38%

2.10 Weight is a measure, not a frequency.

2.11 The frequencies do not add to 100%.

CHAPTER 3

3.1 Ratio; ratio; rate; rate.

3.2 Figure 3.1 graphs a rate (days lost per person per year) by type of worker. A histogram displays a frequency of an interval or class.

3.3 12; 4.

CHAPTER 4

4.1 a) The population is unknown, some women may be counted more than once because of multiple births, repeated confinements.

b) Untreated arthritics may be under-represented.

c) If a sample of registered individuals is taken, large families may be over-represented in the sample.

4.2 A census is necessary only when complete precision is required or when a census costs no more than a sample survey. A small sample may be sufficient if the population is uniformly distributed (e.g., blood sample).

4.3 a) Hospitals.

b) Department heads.

c) All hospital employees in that state at a given time.

4.4 The electrical signals of this patient's heart, perhaps only from a definite point in time.
Because the population is undefined—even if it were defined, it would be impractical to sample at random.

4.5 Representative sample—untrue.

4.6 a) Cheap for the information derived and for its value in planning a full scale study—may be misleading.

b) Can derive confidence intervals of population parameters—may be costly or impractical.

c) Cannot prove cause and effect but may reveal important factors or conditions in the etiology.

d) Useless if the 54% who did not respond did so because of their attitude toward cremation.

CHAPTER 5

5.1 b) 9.12

5.2 Only if both sexes have the same population mean.

5.3 Exclusion of Hopkins is likely to reduce the mean payroll of Maryland hospitals.

5.4 121.1; 122.5; each value is a mode!; 99 to 134; 10.08.

5.5 6 to 10 lbs.

5.6 7, 0.5.

5.7 17/89 = 19.1%.

5.8 Asymmetrical since the median is smaller than the mid-range by about 10% of the range.

5.9 A measure of the variability of the annual crude death rate. The usual graph shows crude death versus time. Histogram shows number of years in which the crude death rate fell in a certain interval.

CHAPTER 6

6.1 1/8 if the "one in the upper quartile" is specified, otherwise 1/4.

6.2 a) $0.10 \leqslant P(\#DMF > 6) \leqslant 0.35$
b) $P(2 \leqslant \# DMF \leqslant 6) = 0.53$
(*Note:* If "between" is interpreted to be "strictly between" then replace $\leqslant$ by $<$.)

6.3 a) *B B G G, B G B G, B G G B, G G B B, G B G B, G B B G*
b) 1, 5, 10, 10, 5, 1
c) *L L L E E, L L E L E, L E L L E, E L L L E, L L E E L, L E L E L, E L L E L, L E E L L, E L E L L, E E L L L.*

6.4 65%.

6.5 63%

6.6 .983, .864

CHAPTER 7

7.1 $74.25 to $86.25.

7.2 25.54 to 38.46; The average increase (or decrease) in productivity of all health care professionals in the system. An apparent increase in productivity which could have been caused by the spotlight effect of the study or an increase in the index but not in actual productivity (i.e., the index may not be a good measure of productivity).

7.3 Confidence intervals are 6 to 35 and 20 to 61.

7.4 $n = 26$.

7.5 191

7.6 Because the confidence level is higher.

7.7 a) $83.10 to $86.90
  b) If $n = 27$, 80% will lie within sample range with 98% confidence. If $n = 31$, 80% will lie within sample range with 99% confidence. Since $n = 29$, we choose the first statement as more conservative.
  c) 5.045, 3.966 to 6.76
  d) i) a, b, c; ii) a, c; iii) a, b, c, except that random selection guarantees independence.

CHAPTER 8

8.1 $6,240 = 13 \times 30 \times 4 \times 4$.

8.2 5

8.3 0.5

8.4 σ may be used to calculate the standard error of $\bar{x}$ as $\sigma/\sqrt{n}$; $\sigma_{\bar{x}}$ describes the sampling variation of $\bar{x}$ in repeated samples of the same size drawn at random from the same population; s may be used to calculate the estimated standard error of $\bar{x}$ as $s/\sqrt{n}$; $s_{\bar{x}}^2$ estimates $\sigma_{\bar{x}}^2$.

8.5 4

CHAPTER 9

9.2 a) Significant
  b) Just not significant.
  c) Not significant.
  d) A random sample from a normal distribution.

9.3 a) Significant.
  b) Not significant.
  c) Same assumptions.

9.4 a) Not significant.
  b) Significant.
  c) As before plus $s = \sigma$.

9.5 a) Not significant.
  b) A two-tailed test based on equally sized samples drawn at random from the (same) normal distribution.

9.6 a) Not significant.
  b) A random sample from a normal distribution.

9.7 Significant evidence of a cycle in this data.

9.8 Not significant.

9.9 Not significant.

9.10 Significant.

9.11 Significant.

9.12 Just not significant.

CHAPTER 10

10.1 Confidence limits of μ are not the same as tolerance limits of a population.

10.2 Disposable sheets

10.3 2, 3, 1 and 5, 4. (Patients 1 and 5 have the same score.)

10.4 Yes.

10.5 $1.89 to $2.71 and $1.76 to $2.84.

10.6 42% to 78%.

CHAPTER 11

11.1 a) Degree of disability.
  b) Height.
  c) Mortality rate.
  d) Average number of office visits per doctor.
  e) Age.

11.2 a) $a = \bar{y} - b\bar{x}$

  b) $a = \bar{y} - b\bar{x} - c\bar{z}$

11.3 a) Significant.

  b) $\hat{y} = 32.82 + 0.608x$

  c) Approximately 61 cents in the dollar.

  d) $32.82 per month.

  e) $83.72

11.4 a) $\hat{y} = a + bx + cw + dv + eu$ where y = time in hours devoted to direct patient care by the professional nursing staff for a given period (say 1 day), x, w, v, u represent factors associated with y, and a, b, c, d, e are the corresponding regression coefficients.

11.5 a) Neither significant. (Note that exclusion of the two outliers permits us to use a linear rather than a quadratic regression.)

  b) 1. 739,696 2. 775,139 3. 739,578 4. 775,015

  c) In all cases, the original data on 51 states.

11.6 Examples of simple time series—a population census repeated every 10 years; the voting preference of an electorate recorded at repeated polls.

Examples of complex time series—the height and weight of an individual over his lifetime; descriptive statistics culled from a series of annual reports for a given hospital over a period of years.

11.7 Significant by the first test, not significant by the second!

11.8

y_t	$\hat{y}_{t+1}$	M.A.
1254	—	—
1234	1254.0	—
1300	1250.0	1293.5
1373	1260.0	1301.9
1280	1282.6	1309.5
1275	1282.1	1313.4
1320	1280.7	1318.5
1384	1288.6	1324.8
1310	1307.6	1328.5
1295	1308.1	1342.4
1330	1305.5	1373.8
1485	1310.4	1386.9
1460	1345.3	1374.4
1250	1368.2	1356.1
1275	1344.6	1323.0
1394	1330.6	1307.4
1286	1343.3	1324.1

1299	1331.9	1331.8
1360	1325.3	1339.0
1370	1332.2	1355.6
1368	1339.8	1370.5
1350	1345.4	1390.9
1428	1346.3	1405.9
1465	1362.7	1405.3
1393	1383.1	1418.0
1380	1385.1	1428.0
1440	1384.1	1439.9
1498	1395.3	1446.8
1490	1415.8	1444.3
1398	1430.6	1464.3
1460	1424.1	—
1520	1431.3	—
—	1449.0	—

where $\hat{y}_{t+1} = .2y_t + .8\hat{y}_t$ and $M.A._t = \frac{1}{8}(y_{t-2} + 2y_{t-1} + 2y_t + 2y_{t+1} + y_{t+2})$

11.9

Day	Period	y_t	D	S_1	S_2	R
1	1	6	6.00	1.00	1.00	0.00
	2	9	6.90	1.00	1.09	0.27
2	1	8	7.42	1.02	1.09	0.34
	2	11	8.46	1.02	1.15	0.55
3	1	7	8.36	.97	1.15	0.36
	2	10	8.70	.97	1.15	0.35
4	1	6	8.20	.90	1.15	0.10
	2	12	8.93	.90	1.21	0.29
5	1	9	9.46	.91	1.21	0.36
	2	12	9.85	.91	1.21	0.37
6	1	10	10.44	.93	1.21	0.43
	2	13	10.83	.93	1.21	0.42
7	1	12	11.76	.95	1.21	0.57
	2	15	12.36	.95	1.21	0.58

(The figures in the above table have been calculated to four decimal places and then rounded off.)

$$\hat{y}_{8,1} = (12.36 + 0.58) \times .95 = 12.29$$

$$\hat{y}_{8,2} = (12.36 + 0.58) \times 1.21 = 15.66$$

11.10

Day	Period	y_t	D	S_1	S_2	R
1	1	6	6.00	1.00	1.00	0.00
	2	9	6.30	1.00	1.04	0.03
2	1	8	6.50	1.02	1.04	0.05
	2	11	6.94	1.02	1.10	0.09
3	1	7	7.01	1.02	1.10	0.08
	2	10	7.30	1.02	1.12	0.11
4	1	6	7.25	1.00	1.12	0.09
	2	12	7.67	1.00	1.12	0.12
5	1	9	7.92	1.01	1.17	0.14
	2	12	8.27	1.01	1.17	0.16
6	1	10	8.57	1.03	1.20	0.17
	2	13	8.96	1.03	1.22	0.19
7	1	12	9.40	1.05	1.22	0.22
	2	15	9.88	1.05	1.25	0.24

(Figures calculated to four decimals and rounded off.)

$$\hat{y}_{8,1} = (9.88 + 0.24) \times 1.05 = 10.63$$
$$\hat{y}_{8,2} = (9.88 + 0.24) \times 1.25 = 12.65$$

11.11 b) 2010

Index